Claireville

A stroll down memory lane

David Fischer MD PhD

DEDICATION

For my mother...

What if the point of life and relationships is not to be happy, but to be holy?
~Regina Bahten, DO

INTRODUCTION

Text, Bubbles: Taylor and I arrive at SMF at 11am. Can we meet in Sacramento somewhere around noon? We leave to Claireville area around 3pm or 4pm.

Bubbles had told me a month before that she was escorting her son, Taylor, to a band competition in Claireville, not far from where I live in Sacramento.

I wanted to see her, but had misgivings.

Me: I was remembering your lovely son Taylor from when I last visited you in Las Vegas 16 years ago. He reminded me so much of you: quiet, introspective, intense. When we went out for breakfast at Denny's and you told the story of your parents appealing to your grandmother for help with Cynthia and what you observed about how cold your grandmother was, I could just imagine Taylor thinking and feeling the same things you did. Naturally, I would like to see him again, just as I'm dying to see you again. But I wonder what you want in that meeting? Whether I could answer any questions he might have about who you are to me? That is, before you were mother to him, I considered you something of mother to me – and, of course, much more. Or whether you would prefer discretion and that I keep to myself the depth of feeling I hold for you?

Bubbles: Wherever talk goes is fine with me.

As the appointed date of your meeting neared, I wondered how I'd be able to contain my feelings for the next days until I got to see

1

her? And what I needed was some time capsule, in which to put myself in hibernation until then.

I wondered what stories I'd tell her son about her? Perhaps, I'd tell him about the time that she pulled me out of the darkest depths of my despair after Professor Hope got so mad at me, and I felt reduced all my scientific aspirations to ashes? Maybe share the poem that I wrote for her after she'd pulled me out of all that, when I'd referred to her as an angel?

Then, a week before our planned meeting, tragedy struck, as I received a call from my brother telling me that my mother died.

Me: I am still in Los Angeles working through the matters pertaining to my mother's passing and sadly will not be in Sacramento to join you and Taylor tomorrow.

Bubbles: I am sad to hear of your Mother's passing. She lived a long life; I'm sure matters can be complicated.

Me: How nice it would have been telling you some stories about my mother.

Bubbles: I would love to hear stories about your Mother someday.

At my mother's house, as well as photos of my mother when she was young, I found the pictures I had taken of Bubbles during our summer together, and looking at them, it felt like I was seeing a different side of her that I didn't appreciate back then; namely, I saw the young, vulnerable, traumatized girl, now along with the very mature young woman.

I arrived back in Sacramento late Friday, so to help those in the long COVID-Qi Gong study and wrote to her the following day.

Me: Happy birthday, Bubbles! I have to treat people with long Covid via Qi Gong for the UC Davis project from 930 until 1130, but after that I'd be happy to drive to Claireville to meet you to celebrate your birthday.

Bubbles: I have the rental so let me know where…

CHAPTER ONE

In Claireville we met at the Starbucks in the Solano Town Center Mall.

I saw her drive in and went to meet her at her car. But it was a while before she opened the door, and looking through the windshield, she looked frozen there.

"Look at you," she said finally opening the door and greeting me.

I responded in kind, telling her that she was as beautiful as ever and hadn't aged a bit. This with greeted with silence. Then, entering the Starbucks, Bubbles commented that she turned 60 today, and a young woman standing next to us in line gushed about Bubbles' youthful appearance.

"I wouldn't have put you a day past forty," she said.

I agreed, though in a short matter of time, I was to learn why perhaps Bubbles didn't...

CHAPTER TWO

A pink lemonade for her and a Frappuccino for me, we walked outside again. She commented she didn't remember when my birthday was? This surprise me, especially since my birthday was essentially an anagram of hers. And I never thought she'd forget my birthday, especially since some years ago, she'd written that she remembered, though stopped sending me cards.

This would be a precursor and theme for much that I would learn that day...

CHAPTER THREE

Heading to the mall, she commented about my text, saying she did not recall me having met her son before and asked when that might have happened? I responded it was 2008 and that I'd met both her sons that day, and especially recalled her husband bounding down the stairs with their infant son, Samuel, introducing him as their "white baby." Then, I was left alone with their toddler, Taylor, who proceeded to pour his cereal on the floor, and later when we went to Denny's, slapped Bubbles on the face.

"He still slapping me on the face," she responded. "Except now he does that with his words..."

I felt sad for her that her son would treat her unkindly, as I'd been at the time of the first slap.

However, even more, I was taken aback that she didn't remember our most recent time together. This was because I had come into our visit with a kind of confidence that I now knew who I was to her. After all these years, I realized now that everything she told me back then was true, and I was someone who she deeply loved. But hearing now that she couldn't even remember our most recent time together, it left me to wonder, "If you can't even remember our last visit together, what can you remember?"

"Right," my best friend, Reuben, would comment later, "because she has made up her life."

"Look," he continued, "you get married to someone, and it's not what you wanted. Or you got married, and you're not in love with that person, but you think, 'This is a good person, and I should marry him because this fits into my plans for my life.'

"So many people get married not because they love each other, but because it fits into their plans. And so the marriage is kind of secondary to their plans, and that becomes a reckoning point in their lives where they're like, 'OK, I can either stick with these plans, or do I reevaluate them and say, 'Maybe this isn't right?'

"Or are they all in? And whether it's right or wrong, they're just going to keep on going down this path?

"And most people tend to keep on going down the path whether it's right or wrong," he concluded. "They don't want to reevaluate…"

CHAPTER FOUR

"I guess it's hard for me to imagine you at the house, because my husband is always talking about how much he hates you," Bubbles said. "And probably the reason why I can't remember the two of you interacting is because I was so stressed and afraid that he would hurt you."

Listening, I lowered my head. I felt sad that her husband would make such comments.

As opposed to her, I had no such fears of her husband – When he came bounding down those stairs and putting his newborn deliberately right in my face with Bubbles watching, I knew exactly what he was doing: He was telling me that by siring Bubbles with children, he had her for good. That he owned her now.

Looking over at Bubbles at that moment, I felt embarrassed for him - That he would stoop to such thoroughly shameful behavior and openly display such a level of pettiness and mean-spiritedness against someone who was obviously suffering, as he was all too aware of the extent to which I loved her.

And I felt sorry her for her that she was bound to someone who would conduct himself this way.

So, when our eyes met at that moment, I felt sure Bubbles knew what he was doing, but was willing to accept her husband's immaturity as a matter of most men being just overgrown "boys."

What I would have never guessed was that she was actually feeling so much fear for me that she wound "check out" and mentally dissociate to the extent that all memory of the events and experiences of that day were lost to her...

"And why would her husband hate you?" Reuben asked later. "Why would it be so important to her husband not to have you in her

5

life? It isn't because of you. It's because of her feelings for you. He's jealous.

"If her husband is jealous of you," he said, "it's because he feels like he doesn't measure up to the love she had for you. If there's an issue, that could be the only issue involved.

"If he felt completely, 100% loved by her, and she was in love with him for who he was and who he actually is and everything about him, he wouldn't be jealous of you. It wouldn't be an issue.

"The only reason why there's an issue is because that issue haunts him… She loves you in a different way than she loves him…. She's never going to love him the way that she loves you.

"And now she has to go through life living with that. And he has to go through his whole life living with that.

"And, so, it's always a question about truth? 'Is this true? Is it not true? Is our relationship true? Is it not true!…'"

CHAPTER FIVE

Bubbles described her husband's upbringing, saying he grew up in Berkeley, where, as a white person, he was in the minority and picked on.

"So, for a long time when we were first together, anywhere we would go and he see a black person, he'd refer to them with the N-word," she said. "And I had to tell him to stop and that wasn't acceptable."

I said my father had all too often used the N-word when I was growing up, and I could never understand how a person from a persecuted minority could speak so badly of another minority?

Bubbles commented that she thought that all minorities should be treated like endangered species.

Yes, treating each other with understanding – That's where real growth could come from.

I was reminded of a conversation I had with my friend, Sam, following the death of my 'soul dog', Ini, who'd begun life as a 'Rez dog' that we'd acquired on an Indian Reservation in South Dakota and blossomed into a source of joy in so many lives.

"Sounds like Newton's law," he said of my relationship with Ini. "'There's an equal and opposite force.' Because as much as you got from Ini, Ini got, as well. It was like an equal exchange of beautiful experiences from both of you.

"It was like you two found each other, though what was neat about Ini was she not only shared herself with you, but with April and anyone else she met and encountered and interacted with. She just had so many capabilities to relate to other beings.

"And I think that's what she did. She was just really open to any other person or animal who came her way."

I'd confided to Sam how it was that as much as Ini enjoyed others, when it came to other dogs interacting with me, she would intentionally get between me and them, as though to say, "No, this is my dad."

Sam acknowledged this, then commented, "But what is selfishness and jealousy? It's thinking that you're going to lose something that you feel is very valuable - Or essential, actually.

"I mean, bad jealousy is one where you're feeling that you're losing something so essential that without it, your life is miserable. And you never know how deep that was?"

"But, the thing that you do know, is all of the things that you experienced with her," he concluded. "So, you're very fortunate that you had that..."

CHAPTER SIX

Just before entering the mall, I asked if I could finish my Frappuccino, because I wanted to wear a mask inside? However, in a short matter of time, Bubbles commented that she was "freezing."

I immediately threw away the drink and escorted her into the mall. Nevertheless, this surprised me because I always remembered her warmth. Indeed, even when I was held by her sister, or her mother, I would experience that kind of warmth from the Vasquez women, and it would remind me of her.

Once inside, she explained she had a propensity for her hands to get cold.

This again would be a precursor to learning about unfortunate aspects of her health...

CHAPTER SEVEN

Walking with Bubbles, I felt all the enchantment that had always accompanied being with her, like the feeling of a totally unexpected gift.

Forty years before, she commented that she thought my looking in those glass windows as we walked was because I was vain... But it wasn't... It was because I was so amazed that this most beautiful of women was walking alongside me.

That feeling of enchantment remains, I thought. She was my first love, and will probably always hold that feeling for me... A deep love that just never ends.

However, whereas I can't forget, I wondered what she remembered?...

CHAPTER EIGHT

I was hoping to purchase her some flowers for her birthday, but not finding a florist, I led her into an art shop, where I was hoping to buy her a present.

Perusing the shop, I was reminded of a painting that I was drawn to years ago with the older, beautiful, brown-eyed woman sitting between a couple of men with their hands at their loins and whose legs embrace a man somewhere out there in the horizon like a spirit against the clouds who holds the key to her heart.

Meanwhile, a photograph of some giraffes caught Bubbles' eye.

She talked about feeding a giraffe, and how it was with their great tongues she was afraid that they wrap their tongue around her hand and swallow her up.

Having seen giraffes in the wild, I was not so impressed and told Bubbles about the experience: It happened while I was travelling in South Africa, and how regal the giraffes were in their family units, the dominant male overseeing the females and the youngsters, walking so elegantly, every joint popping perfectly into place. Indeed, Bubbles, with her great height and wonderful posture, reminded me of a giraffe.

I talked about how it seemed like they were such 'thinking beings', and how much I'd enjoyed all of these creatures I saw were thinking beings, and how much I hated the idea of 'animal farms', like the ones for crocodiles and alligators. These were creatures of the wild who are meant to live by their wits in nature, and not be treated like cattle and farmed.

Bubbles agreed and said it was one of the things that she worried about the world.

I told her about the story of going to South Africa, saying it was because my father gave me tickets good for anywhere in the world, so I asked my friend, Reuben, who had danced everywhere in the world, where could be found the best nature?

"South Africa," he responded, without a second's hesitation.

The shop owner overheard and asked if I was at Kruger Park? I told her no, and that I'd gone to the parks closer to Durban, as I wanted to stay close to my brother, who was surfing on the coast...

CHAPTER NINE

At a Native American shop, the owner tried hard to sell Bubbles some jewelry, but to no avail.

Leaving, she showed me the only pieces of jewelry she was wearing.

"I just wear this silly kid's ring that I just picked up off the ground somewhere and put where my wedding ring used to be, because the wedding ring doesn't fit anymore, because my fingers are becoming all bony because of what the arthritis is doing to them," she said. "My husband keeps telling me to have the ring adjusted, and I say, 'Yeah, yeah', but I just keep wearing this one."

I looked down at my own hand that was without a wedding ring that never felt right on it.

"And this," she added and pulled out necklace with a large, black, accented cross. "My father just said that he wanted a crossed one day. He wasn't religious, but one day he said he wanted one. And this is the one he got. So, I wear it and it gives me comfort, because it reminds me of him...

CHAPTER TEN

She broke down then and apologized for having not informed me about her father's passing and funeral. I told her there was no need for apology and that I could only imagine that, at the time, she was dealing with a thousand things.

But the way she sounded reminded me of all those years ago when she accidentally locked me out of her room...

The next morning Bubbles found out what happened.

"David, I feel so bad..."

"It's okay, Bubbles. It's okay."

She left for a trip to Marineland. I went to my lab and spent the day working on non-extinguishing crystals - a considerably difficult task. I started at 8 am; by 8 PM I was tired, hungry and exhausted, but something inside drove me to keep on.

I came home to find that Bubbles wasn't there. In the bed my mind was filled with apprehensions. Where is she? I miss her. I miss holding her. I miss loving her.

I lay there for hours; trying to sleep, but not able.

Finally, I heard some rustling in the bathroom, then the knob turning.

"Hi Bubbles," I whispered.

"Hi David."

She sat beside me on the bed and told me about her day. Marineland had not gone as well as she'd anticipated. I felt bad for her; I knew how much she was looking forward to it. I sat up in the bed and stroked her face and kissed her forehead.

We talked more about where she went, her long walk, the wind outside.

She undressed and got into bed with me. She curled up next to me and I kissed her and caressed her back with my fingertips until she was asleep.

I was awoken a little later by the sound of her rubbing her eyes. I sat up and stroked her hair.

"David," she whispered, "I feel so bad. I've felt bad all day. I'm so sorry I locked you out. I'm so stupid. I must have locked the door when I went back for my coat. I'm sorry - I'm so bad!"

I kissed her.

"Bubbles, it's okay. I was just glad you were alright because I was worried about you. You're too hard on yourself - I think you're wonderful; you're the most unselfish and caring person I've ever met."

"I don't see how you think that."

"Your actions say that, Bubbles. Look at you - You go to the movies with Stan because you don't want him to be alone - because you're afraid he's lonely and you know you'd be lonely if you were him. You feel bad because you didn't have a place for me to stay one night, when if it weren't for you and your caring I wouldn't have any place to sleep at all."

"I didn't think of those things."

"Once in a while we just need someone to remind us what wonderful people we are."

She reached out her arms and embraced me, holding me and kissing me. Then, she cuddled to me and went to sleep...

CHAPTER ELEVEN

Bubbles commented that I was the only male that her father ever let in the house.

"Well, maybe I'm actually female at heart," I responded. "Just in a male body."

"Well, I always did like the way you walk," she commented. "I guess that does make you female."

I smiled, confused – The 'way I walk' is all twisted from injury, so to resemble the sideways walk of a crab.

And I wondered what she meant by seemingly indicating she like how women walked? Was she attracted to women? She was also the more domineering of the two of us, physically. On one morning during our summer together, as I went about gathering my things, Bubbles caught me in her arms, held me fast, so that there was nowhere I could go, sank her lips against my neck, then crunched through all the tissues there; and in spite of the pain, my reaction was to submit and pull her to me, as though offering myself up to her – even feeling stimulated...

It happened that among my fears about the next life was the thought of coming back as a woman, being that I find the life of women so difficult, especially when I consider the life of my mother and even the woman who stole my mother's husband.

And the thought that Bubbles and I would find each other in different gender states was not reassuring, especially when I considered how much my mother languished over being heartbroken over my father.

But, then, even as a man, I obviously haven't done very well in that department...

CHAPTER TWELVE

She said that she appreciated her time later in life with her father, who she took into her home and cared for when he developed dementia.

"Because even though it was very difficult, and he would get mad and throw glasses full of juice, so that there was broken glass and fruit juice to be cleaned up all over the floor and walls," she said, "I got to see that, really, at his core, he was such a sweet little boy."

"So, it was worth it," she concluded. "To see my father that way..."

CHAPTER THIRTEEN

I talked about how much I loved her father. He was like the father I wanted and never had – who'd converse with me for hours and treat my thoughts and conversation seriously.

And I shared my regret about one of our last conversations, which occurred while I was caring for her mother, just before her mother's heart surgery:

In the early morning Mr. Vasquez stood at the stove preparing breakfast. I sat with him, and he put a plate of potatoes and tortillas on the table for me.

"You need to comb your hair," he said. "There's a right way of doing something and a wrong way, and you want to do things the right way."

I smiled.

"I don't think that it's always that clear cut, Mr. Vasquez," I responded.

"There is always – always – a right and wrong way of doing something," he insisted.

"And what about the shades of gray in between?" I asked. "That cloud and obscure the determination of right and wrong?"

"I'll give you an example," I continued. "While I was in South Africa, I gave a woman a ride. She was colored – of mixed decent – and, for that reason, had a special place in the Apartheid system. She said that she'd been reasonably content with her place in society; but when I condemned Apartheid as an evil, discriminatory state-sponsored system, not different from the Nuremberg laws that Hitler imposed upon the Jews before annihilating them in the Holocaust, it

seemed my words had the effect of 'destabilizing' her – replacing her fragile faith with a cruel reality."

He'd been listening like the gambler he'd told me his father was – with steely eyes that concealed his hand.

"Well, did you do right or wrong?" he asked.

I hesitated, depressing the corners of my mouth.

"I'd spoke the truth, but what I did was wrong," I responded. "If I could do it over again, I would have done it differently."

"That's where you're wrong," he asserted. "You'd done right in the first place. Even if that woman went and blew her brains out after what you told her, you still did right to tell her how things were, because it might have helped her to better her life. You done right and shouldn't think about what she's gonna do – Because you done right."

"You have something wrong with your thinking," he asserted. "Have to change it now or else it get you into trouble."

He shook his head.

"Why you do different with that woman in the car?" he demanded. "Why?"

"Because I scared her," I responded, "and I care about her feelings."

"That's no good!" he countered. "You say that, you say that I don't care about people."

"That's not what I said, Mr. Vasquez..."

"No," he interrupted, "but that's what you're saying."

He got up.

"You have to get straight in your mind," he insisted. "No, 'What about this?' or 'What about that?' Right or wrong – that's it. We shouldn't even be talking about this..."

It struck me that I'd left out perhaps the most significant part of the experience with that woman; that is, how it was she underwent a transformation before my eyes, going from being a motherly-looking figure who I'd offered a ride to bring her home to her children, to being a sexual being for whom there was mutual interest, but no future.

Indeed, at the end of the ride to Durban, she'd become attached to me and relatively distraught: It took the guys I'd befriended at the Indian restaurant to effectively pry her loose from me and get her on that bus and back to her children...

CHAPTER FOURTEEN

Bubbles told me that she preferred boys over girls when it came to offspring.

"Because girls are more mischievous," she asserted.

I responded that when it came to the children of my previous girlfriend (Kate), I loved her boys, and doing things with them like teaching them sports was wonderful; however, being with her daughters, especially her two younger daughters, Alyssa and Ashley, was like being with a couple of angels, and I imagined that it was the same for her mother when it came to she and Libby.

In response, she described how it was that she would annoy her sister by doodling Libby's outward directed "tits", and Edie's inverted nipple.

And it struck me that I'd just seen such doodles in the papers from our time together that I found in my mother's garage?

Going to my phone, I showed her a photo that I'd taken of those things.

"Was this drawing inspired by Libby?" I asked of the torso with oversized breast.

"Yes," she said, excited. "And Edie and the inverted nipple."

Then, it struck me that among the 'mischievous girls' for whom she'd feared the possibility of rearing was herself...

CHAPTER FIFTEEN

I said it was hard for me to imagine her being mean to her sisters.

"Or mean, in general," I added.

But she insisted that she had been. And, worse, she said she would play tricks on her mother, saying that her mother would rely on her to read signs written in English when they go to a store, but that, instead, she'd lead her mother down a path here and there, and how upsetting that must have been when you were relying on someone to guide you.

I shook my head.

"I still can't imagine that your mother didn't regard you as anything less than a pure gift and adored every moment with you," I said. "I remember the way your mother looked at your photo when I was caring for her just before the heart surgery, and she fell in the bathroom…"

Just then, there was the sound of a thump, followed by a loud crash and a woman's voice calling out. Hurrying down the hall I found Mrs. Vasquez laying in a heap on the bathroom floor, Mr. Vasquez already assisting her.

"You see!" he shouted. "She needs surgery!"

We led her to the bedroom.

"I hurt my neck," Mrs. Vasquez cried.

"Can I help?" I asked.

"No!" Mr. Vasquez insisted. "You let her sleep now!"

But she continued to whimper, and Mr. Vasquez appeared at my room.

"You see what you can do," he said.

Cradling her head and neck in my hands, I searched for her cranial rhythm. The rhythm was discordant, as though there were no rhythm at all – only trembling. Finally, I managed to locate something that felt like a pulse and followed it as it migrated from place to place. Following it, I noted that Mrs. Vasquez's muscles were supple and her hair was thin, and again I was reminded of Bubbles.

It was impossible not to notice that her muscles were similar to Bubble's, as was her soft hair. As time passed, the rhythm became more definite. Then, still points occurred, in which the rhythm stopped entirely, signaling her body was healing and undergoing self-repair.

But it was a long process, and, as the minutes ticked by, the sun came out and dusk transformed to dawn, and having nothing else to do, I let my eyes wander about the room until they settled upon the nightstand, on which was a number of children photographs. Studying the faces of the children, I was able to make out the features of each of the Vasquez's spirited daughters – Until I came upon one photo of a little girl who (for the life of me!) I couldn't recognize. And it was odd because her photo was especially encased within a gilded silver frame!

Appearing shy and downtrodden, the girl's hurt eyes were full of tears that looked away from the camera's lens; and a little bird was perched upon her shoulder that seemed to be trying to sing her grief away.

This must be a distant cousin, I speculated, who lives in some impoverished place in Mexico.

Still, I couldn't take my eyes off her, as I experienced some deep-seated feeling of empathy and kinship for her.

Then, I noticed that Mrs. Vasquez was smiling and staring at the photo with me...

"The look on her face, when I was examining that picture of you when you were a little girl with a bird on your shoulder, and I couldn't figure out who that little girl was, and then I turned and saw that your mother was looking lovingly into the same photograph, and when I asked, 'Who is that little girl?', she responded full of joy, 'Bubbles'..."

CHAPTER SIXTEEN

Since about the time I'd known Bubbles, she'd described significant episodes of abuse on the part of her father when she grew up, and it finally occurred to me to ask why and how a strong, upstanding woman like her mother had tolerated it?

She hesitated, then confided that it had got so bad that her mother made plans to leave her father. And when they approached the children and asked who wanted to go with their mother and who wanted to stay behind with their father, Bubbles said she wanted to stay with her father.

This surprised me, considering the abuse that she'd related under him?...

"If I ever cried, he'd thump on my chest and tell me to stop it. I had to suck in my tears..."

"It was because everybody else wanted to go with mom," she said. "And I was afraid that my father would be lonely. So, I said I wanted to stay with him."

"As usual," I thought, just as I had based on her actions from our times in the dorms. "'The angel'"...

CHAPTER SEVENTEEN

We walked around and around the mall, and then I remembered with concern about how tired her feet got the last time we'd taken in a place together.

That was Philadelphia, and I told her I was sorry that I made her walk so much that day.

But she said she didn't mind and appreciated that by walking the way we had we'd got to see the whole city.

I recalled how afraid she got for me when I sat with my legs dangling over the edge of a bridge, and saying she wouldn't do that.

"I guess it's because I've been in some places where people have done bad things," she said.

Yes, there'd obviously been significant trauma in her upbringing.

I thought of her stories about her sister, Melissa...

"My sister, Melissa, got into trouble a lot," she continued. "My father would send me with her to concerts and parties, so that I could watch her and report back to him. We'd get there, and she'd take off with some guy, and I'd be left there all alone with all these strange guys looking at me..."

"She was a wild child," Bubbles said. "Do you remember that photo sequence of her on the wall of the old Bakersfield house? With her making all those faces at the camera?... That was so her. That's how she was."

She said she'd been estranged of her sister and that they had spoken in some time.

Maybe that isn't such a terrible thing, I responded, considering my last interactions with her.

Bubbles looked at me, confused.

24

"What did you say?" she asked.

I repeated myself.

She looked away, as though having difficulty reconciling and apprehending what I'd just said...

CHAPTER EIGHTEEN

We talked about other places we'd gone, like our day in San Francisco, when she got that fortune cookie...

"David, let's go to the Japanese Tea Gardens."

"Alright."

I think we both wanted to hold hands, but walked there separately.

I paid for tickets and we entered the gardens.

I was hungry and bought some fortune cookies. We exchanged fortunes.

"Here's one, Bubbles. 'You will never be hungry.' This one must have been written before I began living in the chem lab."

"I don't like mine."

"What does it say?"

"'You will attain wealth through marriage.'"

"I wouldn't like that one, either."

We passed by a waste basket; she took the fortune out of her pocket, crumpled it up, and threw it away.

"I won't do that next time," she commented of her actions then.

I looked at her.

"When you did that, I think I thought to myself the same thing that Pierre Curie is said to have thought when he met Marie Curie," I said. "'This is a woman of quality'..."

CHAPTER NINETEEN

Bubbles commented that what she remembered about that trip to San Francisco was "getting on the bus and our not having money."

Yes, we didn't have change ready when we got in the bus, so that we had to argue with the driver not to kick us out while I searched my pockets desperately, especially if we were in a hurry to get to her sister, Sylvia, who was already at the wharf waiting for us.

"And then that homeless-looking woman who paid for us," she recalled.

Yes, who knows? I thought. Maybe that 'homeless-looking woman' was an incarnation of my mother, who my brother would often describe as "the bagwoman driving the Mercedes-Benz…"

CHAPTER TWENTY

Walking past a clothing shop, I pointed to a gold ornamental shirt that was not unlike the one I usually on nights that I go dancing or perform karaoke – especially while working on the book about this extraordinary dancer and drag queen, Mercury Rising.

"I just finished that book!" she exclaimed. "It's unusual for me to finish a whole book, because I find I get partway through a book and put it down and pick up some instruction manual or informative something. But your books I always read to the end, because they're so interesting!"

"You've just led such an interesting life, David," she gushed. "You just have. You've done so many things, met so many different people, traveled so many places. You've led such an interesting life."

Then, stepping onto an escalator, I confided that for all of my experiences and things I've done and places I'd traveled, the place where I found the most joy was within the small confines of that tiny room during our summer together.

"In that tiny room, huh?" she responded.

"Yes," I said. "With you…"

CHAPTER TWENTY-ONE

In the summer of 1984, I was inspired to come back to college to continue my x-ray diffraction research. At the time, she was already there, doing an internship at the vet school. I was planning to live in my laboratory, sleeping on the couch there; however, she kindly opened a space on the floor in her tiny dorm room and, in time, we became romantically involved.

Memories of Bubbles in bed beside me, her head nestled against my chest, sleeping together naked in that tiny room represented the happiest moments of my life.

Nevertheless, I was driven then to make my mark in research, so we agreed that this relationship was only going to be for the summer.

But I cherished every moment, such that she became imprinted on me.

Her love was just so pure and unconditional – like nothing that I'd known before or since.

We wound up going our separate ways – me to develop a cancer vaccine, her to become a veterinarian.

But the deep love that she inspired never ends...

CHAPTER TWENTY-TWO

I told her that of my recent experience over the past years, it was my time in the Northern Plains serving native peoples on the Indian Reservations that were probably the most meaningful to me.

I confided about the experience that occurred during my Sweat Lodge ceremony, in which it felt like a spirit had spoken to me:

Intense heat emanated from the stones and permeated the lodge.

"We want to meditate on those who you have come to make this sacrifice," Orville said. "A sacrifice you make in sweat and time."

I thought about the young people who took their lives. Then, I considered the leg injury I'd suffered years before, and the many healing methods I'd been exposed to, and wondered that those experiences might not have prepared me for what I was about to partake in?

"You think you know something. You don't know shit."

It was a voice in my head – yet it came to me so clearly and unlike my own that I turned my head to look around...

I said that I felt that spirit's comment was true, and I didn't know anything about what I was getting into – the historical trauma, etc.

And that those with me in that sweat lodge recognized that I had a gift. I could not only receive and understand messages from the spirits.

And this seem to get around, because I was invited to more and more of these ceremonies, and had more and more meaningful experiences – like the time that during a Sundance when a Medicine Man turned and pointed in my direction, and I experienced a sense

of euphoria, which I intuited as his sending healing energy, for which
I was a bystander...

CHAPTER TWENTY-THREE

When I described my affinity for the Lakota, I said it was because of the 'sanctity for life' that I found in their spirituality.

"For them," I began, "their ways teach that a child born with disabilities represents a spirit whose chose a really difficult path, and for that, they honored that person.

"In contrast, in the home that I grew up in, my father taught this utilitarian view of life, where if you up to his ideals and standards of what was good for something, then you might as well be disposed of.

"And that utilitarian worldview never rang true for me, whereas the Lakota worldview did.

"So, when I found the Lakota spirituality, it was like I had found 'my people'…"

CHAPTER TWENTY-FOUR

Bubbles seemed to resonate with what I told her about the Lakota.

"That sounds like the right way to do things," she said.

She commented that it was her understanding that some tribes were matriarchal in their leadership and asked if it were that way for the Lakota?

I responded that I didn't know, though I'd never heard of a woman chief?

Bubbles asked if in the ceremonies, men and women were treated equally?

I said that I've seen women in the sweat lodge and women participating in the Sundance, though, in truth, women participating in the latter ceremony was relatively rare, and it was more common for me to see them performing flesh offerings.

Nevertheless, in the culture of my adopted spirituality, despite what might be significant gender differences involving participation in their ceremonies, it was my experience that there were more 'woman warriors' than ever...

CHAPTER TWENTY-FIVE

Getting back to the Mercury book, I told Bubbles that, if she'd liked, I could send her some photos from that time with me in a dress.

Then, it occurred to me that she had seen me in a dress before – Her own!

> *In the morning, we got up.*
> *"I like watching you dress, David."*
> *"Thanks. I like watching you undress, myself."*
> *She laughed.*
> *"Okay," she said.*
> *She took off her dress and threw it over me.*
> *I willingly put it on and turned to the mirror.*
> *"It looks pretty good. What do you think?"*
> *"I think you're gorgeous..."*

Really, I just wanted to be naked with her all the time, enjoying her beauty...

CHAPTER TWENTY-SIX

Then, it struck me that she had put on my clothes, too!

"After we went skinny-dipping in Lake Tahoe," I said.

"Yeah, do you remember that picture of me at Lake Tahoe that mom and dad used to keep near the back entrance to the house?" she asked. "Well, I was wearing a purple shirt and navy sweatpants, and I don't think those were mine, because I didn't own clothes like that."

Those photos had graced her family's home for at least 30 years – all the years I'd come there.

"Yeah, I still have them somewhere," she declared. "I just put them away after the house was sold."

I told her that I had not found the album containing the photographs of our summer together and that it appeared my brother had carelessly discarded them from where they'd been in my mother's house.

"What photo do you want?" she asked.

My two favorites were one with the two of us, arm-in-arm, with Lake Tahoe in the background and nature all around us, and the other holding hands in the Berkeley Bell Tower...

CHAPTER TWENTY-SEVEN

Bubbles asked about my relationship with April? I said it really shined in the Venus book she'd just read; we'd had a lot of fun, and I appreciated her wise counsel, as I had when I'd been serving native peoples on the Reservations of the Northern Plains.

I didn't share the horrors that we knew on the Reservation and how they made their way into our lives, so to change them forever; an epidemic that resembled nothing less than a plague; brought forth by an 'evil spirit' that affected one family after another; until all that pain and suffering found its way to our door; and, in its wake, all that was left of our relationship was a partnership, built on trust and mutual respect...

CHAPTER TWENTY-EIGHT

We talked about writing, and she asked about what I considered the difference between writing stories and poems?

"Writing stories, for me, is about honoring the people in my life who have taught me valuable lessons," I said. "Poems, for me, come from God."

I considered sharing a poem I'd recently been inspired to write about her:

On my addiction...

You gave me such an abundance of love
That I still feel it.

You gave me such an abundance of love
That it still fills me.

You gave me an abundance of love
Like nobody else.

Like drugs,
You reset my pleasure setting
Way beyond the normal reading.

So that 40 years later,
Still, nobody has touched it.

Nobody is touching
The joy and the laughter

The connection and physicality
The intimacy and fun.

You are the drug.

She'd told me, "I'll love you forever" – written it on the red napkin I found (still intact!) at my mom's.
Somehow, though, all that had seemed to transfer to me.
It was like the poem said - I wound up addicted.
The vast majority of the homeless Veterans I currently served had problems of addiction. I'd even acquired Board Certification in Addiction Medicine. However, all that experience and book learning paled in comparison to the degree to which Bubbles had taught me what it was to have an addiction.
I mean, let's face it, like a recovering drug addict, I craved being with Bubbles every day.
The last time we got together was some 16 years ago. That was when I visited her in Las Vegas after the birth of her children. When I was working on the cancer vaccine, I met her in Philadelphia. That was 30 years ago. And what did we do? We explored the city of Philadelphia together, and at the end of the day, I departed and we went our separate ways.
I took a wife. I've had wonderful relationships with friends and coworkers; I'm a highly productive member of society. And I've had lovers.
However, in time, being in love with others has always come and gone.
But it never left with her.
Walking around the Claireville Mall, every moment felt enchanted. Being with Bubbles delivered a certain quantum of dopamine to my system that's different: When I walk with her, I'm on Cloud Nine. Just the degree of enchantment I feel... I bathe in....
Just to walk along her side...

CHAPTER TWENTY-NINE

Finally, she suggested that we sit at a bench.

"I've been meaning to ask you," she began. "What did you mean when you said that it bothered you to be farther away from me?"

This referred to my impending plans to take a position at Yale in Connecticut.

I hesitated and considered how best to answer.

"I thought it meant that you wouldn't be able to sense my energy," she inserted.

No, I responded. It wasn't that. I didn't particularly think that extending the radius of the Qi field an extra couple thousand miles would make that kind of difference – This based on my experiences in 'remote healing', as well as the teaching of Qi Gong masters:

"Because Chi works on a purely energetic level," one Chi Gong healer commented, "the distance between the practitioner and the client is not a limiting factor, as energy is not restricted by space or time. In fact, certain people respond better to distant healing treatments than to in-person sessions."

What bothered me was that, at present, we were both living on the West Coast, so that if she was ever to invite me to do something, there was a more than reasonable chance of me joining her.

"Like today," I said. "Whereas if I were on the East Coast, it would be more difficult."

"Even though I haven't seen you for 16 years, I'm always hoping that I will," I continued. "And I'll drop everything to do it, given the opportunity. And it will be more difficult when I'm all the way on the other side of the country.

"I don't want to be further from you. I want the opportunity to drop everything and spend time with you…"

CHAPTER THIRTY

She responded that perhaps her son would go to college in Ohio, and then she would visit him, and perhaps we could meet there on the East Coast?

She talked about her son for a while, saying that of the schools they looked at for him, she was most impressed by the students at USC, and found other places like UCLA more ostentatious, relying on mostly their prestige and reputation...

CHAPTER THIRTY-ONE

"Do you think you're kind of stuck?" she asked intentionally.

Lowering my head, I told her, yes, and that I thought she was right. I was 'stuck'. There had not been closure in our relationship.

And it was me to blame for perhaps not having looked hard enough for someone to replace her, or perhaps it was just because people would enter my endorphin system and then leave it, and the problem was that she never left, so it was always her I was coming back to.

Or that I loved her more than anyone? Whatever it was, I thought about her every day...

CHAPTER THIRTY-TWO

I described my confusion at the time of our parting, how it was that I was caught between my drive for cancer research and the feelings that she'd awakened; I was trying to get back to just doing my work as I had before, but that I would miss her, and then try to bury my chest pain in my books and my studies; and that I regretted ever pushing her away, because she didn't deserve that - she only deserve my appreciation.

"We were on different paths," she responded.

Yes, but our paths crossed, I replied, and I wasn't the same after that. She had taught me that life was more than just meaningful work. That's the best part of life was the fun and joy that people could share with each other.

It struck me how traumatized I was: I went from that tiny room in which I shared a relationship of pure bliss with Bubbles, to being stuck in that dark apartment with nothing but a blank wall in front of me, crouched over my books, and all the time missing Bubbles.

"It manifested in confusion, and you didn't deserve that," I said. "You showed me that beyond working towards a calling in life, there was joy that makes life worthwhile. And the most joy I ever experienced was with you..."

CHAPTER THIRTY-THREE

Bubbles expression changed and darkened, as she shared her thought that the word 'woman' might have come from women being "the woe of man."

I listened, because I wanted to be present for her. Though, later, I would wonder if I had any role in such thoughts, and castigate myself for having not reminded her of what I'd told her in a dream years ago – That she was to me 'God's greatest gift'...

CHAPTER THIRTY-FOUR

She offered a string of questions about life on the planet... How it was that life on the planet was just too hard?

It made me think about her father that evening in the treehouse:

As well as me, Mr. and Mrs. Vasquez were entertaining his older brother, Juan. Juan was a born-again convert, and held strong opinions on the matter of faith and religious doctrine. There was the usual banter, but, suddenly, Mr. Vasquez's face twisted in rage.

"If there is a God, I say, 'I curse You! I curse You!'"

"No, Chavo," Mrs. Vasquez interceded, trying to calm him.

But her attempts were to no avail, as Mr. Vasquez's expression only darkened.

"I curse Him!" he continued. "That my daughter, Sylvia, can't have children – That she had to have that operation. I say to Hell with Him! I curse Him!..."

And then the obituary that I'd written for him.

Mr. Vasquez took in this lonely boy when I was twenty.
He taught me so many lessons.
Gave me so much of his time.
He was more than a father...

He loved his family.
When his wife collapsed in the bathroom
And lay in a heap on the floor,
He lifted her with his bare hands,
And saw to it that she got the care she needed

44

That saved her life...

He loved his daughters – and would invite the wrath of God rather than accept anything but a full life for them!...

Courage – That's what he had in abundance.
The courage to speak his truth at every moment.
I suppose that's what one earns
When he's "Never backed down from a fight."

Ultimately, Mr. Vasquez was a towering figure of compassion.
"When you're a doctor," he told me, "and an older couple comes to you asking for medicine, and you take care of them and you charge them a dollar, and all they have is 90 cents, you give 'em a break. Give 'em a break..."

In my mind's eye I see him in Heaven
Arguing for more compassion
For His/Her creations
With God...

CHAPTER THIRTY-FIVE

Then, Bubbles raised other questions like was there really evolution?

"What was the proof?" she asked.

I said I'd written about comparative evolution in my book, The Bioenergy School of Medical Chi Gong:

Addiction, Medical Chi Gong & the Brain

So, let's take an even deeper dive into 'the mind' so to attempt to better understand addiction and the 'energies' involved. Experts in the field of addiction have regarded patients in the throes of addiction as being guided by their 'reptilian brain.' To understand what's meant by this, let's review MacLean's Triune Brain hypothesis.

In the 1960s, American physician and neuroscientist Paul D. MacLean proposed the 'Triune Brain' as a model of the evolution of the vertebrate forebrain and behavior. It can be viewed like this:

1. In the beginning, there was only the reptilian brain, which belonged to reptiles and birds and produced thoughts that were limited to instinctual behaviors that involved in aggression, dominance, territoriality, and ritual displays;

2. Later, with the evolution of early mammals came the paleomammalian brain (paleo- meaning 'old'), such that to the basal ganglia was added the components of the limbic system (namely, the septum, amygdalae, hypothalamus, hippocampal complex, and cingulate cortex), which guided the motivation and emotion involved in feeding, reproductive behavior, and parental behavior;

3. Finally, with the evolution of 'higher' mammals (especially humans) came the addition of the cerebral neocortex, conferring the ability for language, abstraction, planning, and perception.

Hence, the triune brain model proposes that we humans have all of these brain structures (reptilian brain, limbic system and cerebral neocortex) which usually act together, but can act relatively independent of each other. To break it down again: 1. The reptilian brain is in charge of our primal instincts; 2. The limbic system is in charge of our emotions; and 3. The neocortex is responsible for objective or rational thoughts.

That's how addictionologists can assert that the thoughts and actions of patients in the throes of addiction are governed mostly by their 'reptilian brain.' All that matters to them is survival – such that when they are physiologically withdrawing from drugs (whether they be in the class of opioids or amphetamines or alcohol), all that matter is their survival (which comes down to getting that next 'fix'). In between, these patients are typically guided by the next level of brain function (i.e., the limbic system), such that everything comes down to emotional displays for getting more of the drug. It's only when they reach the higher levels of recovery that they really engage their neocortex and come around to understanding what had been driving their behaviors, arrive back at rational thought, and literally have the opportunity to come back to their humanity.

So, finally, how does all this relate to Medical Chi Gong? Consider the chakras/energy centers: As previously asserted, in general, it would appear that the lower chakras are primarily responsible with maintaining survival and function at the reptilian brain; the middle chakras with managing our emotions and function at the level of the limbic system; and the higher chakras with connecting us to our 'higher selves' (which involves altruism, selflessness and spirituality) and function at the level of the neocortex. When I perform Medical Chi Healing, I typically feel an activation of the crown chakra. Is this because Medical Chi Gong is mostly guided at the level of the neocortex (which represents the highest level of our brain function) and then helps coordinate the healing activity (frozen release, etc.) promoted and facilitated by the other parts of our brain? Again, I believe these are questions about this practice for which science is needed to fathom...

I'd previously shared the following thoughts in my book about Ethel...

"I suppose I look at life from an evolutionary point of view, Ethel. In the beginning, there were unlimited resources, and organisms flourished. Now, those resources are dwindling, and if we are to survive as a species, we must find another source of energy - One that is not only recyclable, but, also, self-propagating. The only source of energy I know like that is love. When you love someone, it grows and snowballs and spreads one to another. That's where I think our hope as a species lies..."

My therapist would later comment, "What? She doesn't believe in evolution?... It's hard to be with someone like that."

But I dismissed her disparaging comments, saying that evolution was a 'theory', and who was I to judge?...

CHAPTER THIRTY-SIX

My sadness and heartache went away as I listened, and I looked upon her smiling.

I wanted to tell her that she certainly was no "woe of man" to me – As I'd told her in a dream, "You are to me God's greatest gift…"

In general, it felt like Bubbles was on a search to understand things that were important for her to know.

This wasn't the person who was all about me 40 years ago - This was a person who was on her own quest.

And what she needs is a friend, I decided. Someone in her corner – like what my mom needed and mostly didn't have.

"Is it centered upon the conflict between science and religion?" April asked later.

Whatever it was, it was hers, and I just wanted to be there to support her?…

CHAPTER THIRTY-SEVEN

She described difficulties at her place of work of 30 years, where she felt terribly unappreciated, typically passed over by male coworkers and counterparts, and treated in a disrespectful manner.

She admitted that she wondered if she had done the right thing with her life? Staying and working with this company? Even students she had trained when they were in high school, she got to watch be hired at higher salaries and better benefits than hers.

"What do I have to do?" she asked. "Quit and then reapply? I don't want to quit. I don't want to leave my clients."

I told her that I was sorry that she was being mistreated, and for the life of me I could not understand how anyone would mistreat someone like her?...

CHAPTER THIRTY-EIGHT

She talked about the difficulty of taking care of her population, which was typically underprivileged, and how it was she often felt the sting of 'kill the messenger' when it came to delivering bad news about the high cost of pet care, saying some had been abusive towards her and even threatened her.

Again, it was hard to imagine such a beautiful person being treated that way.

But that said, given how important Ini was to us (and even with the resources that we had, we didn't always want to pay out with the Veterinarian's were asking), I couldn't imagine what it was for these poor people...

CHAPTER THIRTY-NINE

She said she hadn't given her children a fun enough childhood and felt bad that she'd never taken them to Disneyland.

"I could just see that being one of a list of things they'd say while laying on the psychologist's couch," she said.

She added that she felt she was a relatively unsympathetic mother.

"I tell them, 'If you're going to do crazy stuff and hurt yourselves, I'm not spending all night with you in the emergency room. I'm just going to glue you up myself.'"

I tried to reassure her that she didn't have to worry.

"Look at me," I said. "I just feel love for you…"

CHAPTER FORTY

"You said that I had been something of a mother to you," she said. "I didn't remember that in our relationship. What made you say that?"

I could recounted numerous examples – Like when she bought me that toy sword in Chinatown, or when she would come around with her picnic basket and bring me bagels for lunches when I didn't have anything to eat at the lab. When she'd cover me with a blanket when I'd fallen asleep without one. And the experience of drying me after a shower...

We showered.
When we finished, I turned off the water, and she took the towel.
"First, your hair," she said, running the towel through it.
"Then, you scalp. Then, your eyebrows.
"Then, your nose - The whole towel!
"Your shoulders - Lift your arms, cutie!
"Your arms and underarms. Your chest, your stomach, your belly button...

Whereas, when it came to my mother, I only remembered times that if I ever got out of the shower and there wasn't a towel and I was cold and called for my mother, she came begrudgingly and took her time.

And, per her accounting, maybe Bubbles had been like that to her children, and it was just me who got to experience her as a sweet mother, to make up for the one I never had.

"It sounds like I came around at the right time in your life," she said.

You did, I said. Though I couldn't imagine a 'wrong time' for her to 'come around'...

"She was a person who saw you with unconditional love," Reuben would comment later. "Who just saw you, and loved what she saw - Big nose and all.

"And she loved that way. Her heart was open to you. And your heart was open to her.

"But, Mike, you've got to realize... And she probably realized it, too... You were married to something else.... You were married to a life path that you had been living... That has driven you.

"Because I knew you, and we were close when you and Bubbles were close. I know at that time your biggest reservation was that you had places to go and you had to be alone. You knew it. And she knew it. Because she saw all of you. And she knew that where you were going, she couldn't go..."

CHAPTER FORTY-ONE

She said that I could thank her mother for the sweet, caring ways that she showered on me.

I said that I had hoped that I had been able to thank her mother in my attempts to help when I did.

"You did!" she cried. "Mom would always be talking about you, coming and helping and what a difference it made..."

CHAPTER FORTY-TWO

I told Bubbles it was my opinion that my mother froze to death in her own home as a result of the furnace not working.

"It sounds like she decided that it was just time to give up," Bubbles responded.

Yes, my brother had said something to that effect – That my mother was refusing to pay bills...

Later, when I shared Bubbles' comment about "giving up" with April, April commented, "That's what we were kind of hoping for with Ini."

Yes. With Ini, as ill as she was, she refused to give up. Indeed, to the last moment, she would endure anything for another moment to give more love. Perhaps, because she was so loved that she wanted to go on living in spite of everything (Which didn't make me feel better about my mother).

"And with your mother, it was different," April added. "Because all she needed was a little bit of heat. And your brother and nephew should have been able to give her that. If they did, she would probably still be with us..."

Returning to the conversation with Bubbles about my mother, she concluded simply, "It sounds like she picked the wrong son to take care of her..."

CHAPTER FORTY-THREE

I told Bubbles about the unfair way my mother felt she had been treated: My grandfather rejected her pleas to be a part of the family business, insisting that she was a girl and her role was to be a housewife and bear children; my father saddled her with two children before leaving her for a topless dancer. She had no one in her corner. Only perhaps a little boy who did the best he could to be a therapist and source of support, until he went off to college.

Now, all these years later, I can understand why my mom was so rattled when grandpa had that heart attack of his - It was because my grandfather, in spite of all his flaws for being amount to a 'man of his time' (which he was when it came to his antifeminism) had kept my mother and us afloat. He was generous. He wouldn't let her fall and just die.

And when she lost him, she basically lost that support. She lost that net that was under her and been left with nothing to keep her safe.

And it seemed to me that if you don't have somebody in your corner, you're finished – Then, you don't have what it takes to get through this world.

We all need someone in our corner.

Because when you're alone in this world, without a friend or hand to hold or source of support, you might as well check out...

CHAPTER FORTY-FOUR

Returning to the subject of my mom's death, I described how she was found: She'd died in her bedroom in the same place as her favorite dog, Muffin.

However, whereas Muffin died in her dog-bed in a warm home, my mother died on the floor in an unheated house.

In response, Bubbles clearly grasped the moment.

"It sounds like she died worse than a dog," she said....

CHAPTER FORTY-FIVE

Bubbles excused herself, and complained about needing to use the restroom frequently, as a middle-aged woman who'd bore children.

Watching her trot off, her step had its familiar 'bounce', but she was walking on the edge of her feet.

She'd spoke disparagingly about her physical appearance, saying that her abdomen was all bloated.

But her legs were shapely, and I watched her, admiringly....

CHAPTER FORTY-SIX

Bubbles indicated that she wanted to walk again.

I asked if we could go back to the photograph store, so that I could gift her a photo from there?

But she declined, saying her home was already overcrowded, with clutter and lack of wall space.

"And, anyways, it's usually better when I don't get something, because, that way, I keep it in my memory and it stays on my mind..."

I wondered if I wasn't that way with me? This person who she knew and now keeps in her memory, just like that photograph of the giraffe that she'd prefer to keep in her head than purchase and try to find a space for it in her overcrowded home, which was too crowded for me or anything...

CHAPTER FORTY-SEVEN

In a relatively vacant area of the mall, we found a Giant Adirondack Chair.

She got in first, then invited me to join her with a wink.

Climbing in and sliding beside her, I put my arm around her shoulder, like she'd done with me during our trip to San Francisco.

For a moment, it felt as though life had gone full circle; but unlike me forty years ago, when she'd broken through this shy boy's walls, it was as if she were armoring herself, constructing a wall or mental barrier to shield herself from feeling and opening herself to too much, and I withdrew my arm...

CHAPTER FORTY-EIGHT

Still seated on the giant chair, I looked down at her exposed ankle, which she had told me that she had injured last month and was still bothering her.

"I was stupid," she'd said. "I was trying to walk upstairs on my tippy toes, thinking it would help with the jazz dancing, and I slipped and twisted it."

Thirty years before, she'd found cranial sacral therapy helpful, so I offered to perform that now.

Positioning myself behind her, I placed my hands on either side of her head and followed her cranial rhythm, which was even and regular.

"Bubbles, put your hands on mine and see if you don't perceive the movement," I said.

She lifted her hands and gently pressed them to mine.

"Do you feel that?" I asked.

"Yes, I do," she said.

Just then, the rhythm stopped, and in its place came a chaotic release of spasms that felt like a lot of undulating worms under my fingers.

Still point, I thought. But that's something that happens when there's a problem? There's no problem here.

Slowly, her cranial rhythm returned.

"I wonder why that happened?" I commented, confounded.

"I'd been having a stomachache before we started," she responded. "I don't have a stomachache anymore."

She smiled.

"I'm proud of you, David," she said. "I'm proud of what you're doing with your life."

"But isn't that something that you do on someone's head?" she asked. "How can you do that on my ankle?"

I said that although the cranial sacral rhythm originated from the head, it could supposedly be perceived everywhere in the body, and perhaps we could give it a try?

She removed her ankle brace and asked if she should take off her socks?

I told her that I thought she could keep her socks on.

But when she took off her shoes, I wished I had asked her to take her sock off; because under her socks, the outlines of her feet looked nothing less than crippled and shriveled.

No wonder she went quiet with that young woman who complimented her about her youthful appearance, I thought. Because, inside, she's dealing with conditions like atrial fibrillation and crippled feet!

"The feet have the greatest wear in your body," my friend, Sam, would comment later. "You are walking on them, running on them, pounding on them all the time. So that's going to accelerate their change more than any other body part."

"And, the other thing is, people don't observe their feet very often," he added. "They're kind of hidden way down there. I think that's the reason why many diabetics have their feet amputated. Because they're just not paying attention to them...."

Yes, she was probably paying attention to everyone and everything else, and not herself.

As for me, I felt ready to cry at the state of them.

"So, does she have love in her life?" Reuben would ask later. "Or has she decided to live a life of just, on the surface, everything looks good, but, underneath, it's all rotten?..."

Although I have never attempted it before, I immediately perceived her cranial sacral rhythm at her ankles! And not long after, still points occurred.

"I'm feeling twitches in my legs," she said.

Yes, I responded. This was the stage at which healing occurred...

CHAPTER FORTY-NINE

Bubbles asked how I taught Qi Gong to the folks in my research project?

I told her about the self-practice that I had developed, and that it was based on my experience following caring for her mother.

When my work was done and it was time to leave Bubbles and her family, I was expecting it to be as difficult as it always was (because I loved them so much). Hence, stepping onto that departing Greyhound bus and taking a seat in the back, I drew a deep breath and wondered, 'When is it going to hit? The remorse and sadness?'

Then, as the bus drove off, I became aware of an emerging feeling: It wasn't the familiar emptiness and hollowness in my chest, but, rather, a sensation of energy, starting at my head till beaming and overflowing to every part of me, so that I was enveloped in a cocoon of energy, fuller and more expansive than anything I'd ever experienced before!

'I've honored something,' were the words that came to me. 'I've shown some great respect. It's something simple, yet wonderful. It reaches to the core of my being – God is love...'

And that's what I was feeling now as I worked with K remotely, leading me to believe that (more than anything else) what K needed to facilitate healing was to release the retained energy of trauma associated with troubled, trauma filled world of his childhood by tapping into and connecting with the universal energy of love.

Ultimately, Bubbles and I got to attempting the tangibility exercise again, and unlike 30 years ago, this time she was able to perceive energy - Not only over my hand, but also my forearm!

"I feel heat," she said. "It's like squishing a ball."

I shared the story of training and "exercise" to achieve Chi perception, as, again, from my book, The Bioenergy School of Medical Chi Gong:

What if you're one of the 10-25% of people who doesn't perceive points of energy in the Tangibility Exercise? What then? Does it mean that you're just never going to learn BioEnerQi?

To answer this question, I want to begin by sharing an experience involving my car.

This story begins on a day that I was playing tennis with my friend, Danny. After our game I invited him to lunch. He responded that he'd like that, but his car was in the shop. So, I offered to drive.

But no sooner had we pulled out of the parking lot than he told me, "Mike, you got a bearing problem. Don't you hear that 'Rr rr rr' sound?..."

Danny had worked for Ford Motor Company, so I immediately took the car to the mechanic. The mechanic agreed. Indeed, he immediately assessed that the problem was so severe that he was afraid to so much as test drive the car around the block for fear that the wheel assembly would fall off!

The thing is, though – I never heard the bearing problem. Indeed, I'd been driving the car 70-miles every day, commuting between work! Over a bridge no less! Considering the circumstances, that chance invitation to Danny to let me drive him to lunch might have saved my life.

The point is, when it came to my car's bearing problem, I chalked up my inability to hear the defect as a matter of some people being more mechanically inclined than others (like me). In turn, I thought it was the same with energy perception: Some of us can perceive points of energy, whereas others can't.

But others have challenged that assumption.

"I think if you would have practiced, you would have been able to hear the problem bearing," a colleague asserted. "I bet you can become very sensitive to these mechanical issues if you train for it. You just didn't have that experience long enough to train yourself to be aware of that abnormality."

"So, I bet most people – 98 or 99% – can learn to experience Chi," he concluded.

And this does agree with my observations: Even those who begin with minimal perception of energy points are able to advance to greater energy perception with time, training and practice. Furthermore, some who were not able to perceive energy in the tangibility exercise were later able after they'd taken up Tai Chi...

CHAPTER FIFTY

"I think the reason I didn't feel it before was because I didn't believe it," she said. "But now I've had experiences with animal energies, so that I can believe it, and I'm more open."

I confided how much I'd enjoyed watching her interact with animals, even back 25 years ago when I visited her at the pet hospital. Indeed, it was so inspiring so to lead me to aspire to interact with my patients that way and motivated much of my desire to bring Qi Gong into the exam room, because connecting with the energetic circulation always slows me down and inspires me to be more caring.

Later, though, I wondered how it could be that she didn't believe in Qi? Afterall, thirty years ago I had taken care of her mother using Qi Gong? She'd literally helped pay for the plane ticket, so that I could come out there from DC? Why would you not believe?

And even if you didn't believe, could you block yourself enough so to get in the way of feeling?

Then, I considered an example from my own life, when a beloved uncle punched me in the solar plexus, and instead of registering the experience with a feeling of pain, I just registered being without air.

In retrospect, I think I was so unwilling to believe and recognize that my uncle had done this, that it interfered with my ability to register the sensation of pain involved in the experience. I just loved this person so much that I blocked what he had done to me; I was so invested in that emotion of loving my uncle that I wouldn't let myself register the pain involved.

"That's understandable," my father had told me. "When you have trust in an individual, and then that trust is betrayed, it can be difficult to take in the very real message that, 'This relationship is not healthy for me. This person is harmful to me.'"

So, I knew from experience that emotion could short-circuit my perception of feeling.

"It's a form of not accepting what's being offered because you don't believe it can be beneficial," my father had said.

And then I realized that's what probably happened with Bubbles... And I felt I knew exactly when: It was after the winter break following our summer together; I saw her on the quad and invited her back to my place, and told her about my evening with Reuben's lovely sister, Nancy, which culminating with me holding her.

I was just doing what I used to when we were friends.

But she was no longer just a friend. She was bonded to me. She might have gone back to her old boyfriend, but I couldn't be with a new girl.

Because she was my girl. Just like the way it was with Ini.

As a result, she felt hurt and betrayed.

"I love you," I told her, as she moved to leave my apartment that last time.

"No," she mouthed, subtly shaking her head – Too traumatized to speak.

She even told me as much: When next we met in the basement of the library to get together to celebrate my 21st birthday, she said, "My sister says that people who love each other just want to hurt each other. What do you think?"

No, I'd responded, confused. I think people who love each other want to help each other.

But that's what she thought – She felt betrayed. That's probably why she hadn't been open to bioenergy back then – Because I'd betrayed her trust, and she was justifiably wary of my energy...

Postscript:

About a year later, I broached the subject of animal energy experiences with Bubbles again, and she responded as follows:

"I wouldn't say that I have experiences of feeling energy," she began. "It's more like I sit with a group of people in a house of worship, and I start to feel this energy come into me from my palms. It just feels so warm.

"And when I'm with animals, I don't know if it's truly energy or what it is? Maybe it is a sensing of energy? The same as when you sense good situations and bad situations around us? A sence that something's wrong and maybe I should go to the other side of the street? Something?

"Because, for me at least, these animals – they come in with their owners, quiet, mean, sad, whatever it is – and I'm able to sit there calmly and start speaking to them, and they relax, and then they act different, until the owner says, 'All right, it's time to go', and then their posture changes all of a sudden.

"And one thing my sister, Silvia, said to me before was like, for her, she felt it was more some sort of telecommunication. Because she said her dog taught her how to sense communication from others. She said she was just able to talk with her dog in her mind, she felt. And feels like she can harness that same sort of energy like with other animals and with people.

"So, it's different. It's not like I sense heat or anything. It's usually just more an anxious energy."

"I never felt like I doubted you had the sense of feeling energy," she concluded. "I just like feel I can't command it..."

CHAPTER FIFTY-ONE

Bubbles asked if I had energy experiences with animals? I told her about the following experience with Ini, described in my BioEnerQi Handbook:

Massive resets.

It is my experience that massive resets can happen with Medical Chi Healing alone. Case in point is my dog, Ini: Ini developed a condition called Granulocytic Meningomyeloencephalitis (GME), a condition whereby the immune system attacks the nerves throughout the body, resulting in generalized pain, fever, incoordination, seizures and depression for weeks, with most dogs not surviving it.

Fortunately, we found a veterinarian who specialized in Neurology and Neurosurgery, who pulled Ini through; however, even after her condition was stabilized with immunosuppressants, Ini was still racked with pain. Her nerve endings had been effectively fried everywhere. Indeed, people who suffer from something equivalent to her condition (like arachnoiditis) usually require massive doses of steroid and narcotic medication to tolerate the associated pain.

Then, later, when Ini was referred to an Integrative Medicine specialist who learned about my expertise in Chi Gong, he suggested I perform Medical Chi Healing on Ini.

For weeks I did this on a daily basis and saw no change in Ini's condition. Then, one day, after performing Medical Chi Healing, Ini's whole body looked to be doing the equivalent of 'the wave.' It wasn't anything like the typical twitches and fasciculations that accompany a dog's sleep; rather, her whole body was moving like a sine wave – VOOM! VOOM! VOOM! – over and over again. It was as though some switch had been flipped and the result was this massive reset that involved every muscle in her body – contracting and relaxing in one major wave after another.

And when the process was through, she was a different dog: she could tolerate being petted, which she hadn't before because the nerves have been so sensitized; she could tolerate heat or sunlight, which she hadn't since the start of the condition; and she was relatively free of pain!

"She not only came back from the dead," a colleague commented. "She turned into a pup. Your slow process of addressing one problem at a time, doing Medical Chi Healing every day, led to that massive reset. Because then all of a sudden everything just snaps together. It's like spontaneous combustion. It's like how we evolved. There was this primordial soup and then the molecules just came together. But it took years and years. It was a slow process. But then once it matched up, then it was just like an explosion – BOOM! – and then things quickly accelerate and suddenly start happening.

"I think that's the way our body works, too. We just slowly ascend so we don't over pressurize from a dive, but then when we reach the surface, we breakthrough..."

"Did she expand on what she experienced with animals?" April asked. "Did she perceive energy from animals?"

I don't know, I said. I didn't ask.

"It would be interesting," April responded. "To hear those stories..."

CHAPTER FIFTY-TWO

I took Bubbles through the self-practice, although she was mostly wanting to just perceive the energy at her hands, which I told her was fine at her level.

She called me a pioneer in this field. But she has been with me throughout this journey.

She asked how often she should receive these treatments?

"When should I be treated next?" she asked.

When you need it, I answered. With my friends, like Sam, I would usually meet with him at his house once a week.

She said that her ankle felt better, and that the range of motion was improved, so that she didn't want to put the brace back on.

But I reminded her about the mistake we made the last time, when I suggested that she didn't take her asthma medication after we worked on that energy disturbance at her chest, and said that I didn't want to see us repeat that mistake, and told her I thought she should put the brace back on.

Still, walking, she made it very clear to me that her ankle felt better.

I wanted to reach out and hold her hand then and considered the lifetime of the energetic experiences between us: The day I left her family after caring for her mother before her heart surgery, and expecting to feel my usual sadness and remorse at the thought of not having made a life with her so that they were family and my relations, and, instead, experiencing that extraordinary feeling of connecting with the energetic circulation in a way like I never had before, so it felt like there was this energy cocoon all around me, and a feeling of euphoria, and acknowledgment and affirmation that "God is love."

And the feeling that that happened because of her sending energy to me – because she was happy with me and appreciated that I'd helped her mother.

In general, it seemed that my interactions with her had all had some aspect of having been at an energetic level. That they came from feelings that emanated from her heart. If they don't emanate from there, there isn't the same energy experience.

And I can perceive energetically when she was blocking her feelings.

I suppose that my energy experiences with her were the most distinctive and definite because the relationship with her was the most significant of my life – when I totally lost myself in another human being – when I totally gave myself to another.

Indeed, when I recall the times when we were intimate, the only memory that really surfaces was the look of serenity on her face that shone through the night like a light in the darkness, and then being held by her. In other words, it was spiritual.

Forty years ago, she opened me to the energetic circulation, and that experience during our picnic lunch was an energy experience.

On a summer day my beloved college friend Bubbles and I rode out to the fields beyond the campus, and sitting under the shade of a tree sharing a picnic lunch, exchanged stories from our lives. She described the sad occurrence of a neighborhood girl struck by a drunk driver; the girl had been riding her bike at the time, and when she died, Bubbles' father reacted harshly.

"He took our bikes away," Bubbles said. "We were never allowed to ride them again."

She broke off and looked away. Gazing at her I knew her father had only acted to try to protect the daughters he loved! But, at the same time, I realized it made her sad.

Then, it happened: I forgot myself and all that mattered was my cherished friend; and in that moment, I had a feeling like I'd left my physical body and were existing only in spirit.

"I feel for you," I said, reaching out to her. "I feel for you..."

I didn't find that feeling again until I encountered bioenergy. Then, connecting with the energetic circulation, it was like, "Hey, this is what I felt that day under the tree with Bubbles."

When I look back to that moment, I think that it derived from the fact that, first, she gave me unconditional love, and then I felt it for her, and that's what lay behind the bioenergy – at least, for me...

CHAPTER FIFTY-THREE

Returning to the subject of her asthma attack from all those years ago, I told her that I was sorry, and had learned from the experience, and not repeated the mistake.

She accepted my apology.

"Yeah, I hate that," she said. "When you advise somebody about their medications and it doesn't work out right."

Still, it struck me as odd now: Where I now knew she hadn't believed in Qi Gong at the time, why had she even entertained going without her asthma medication then?

Ultimately, I decided that I didn't have a clue?

At worse, it sounded like she was looking for a self-fulfilling prophecy that the bioenergy treatment wouldn't work and her condition would flare?

But that night taught me something else – I learned firsthand how she'd suffered under her father and got a glimpse of how traumatic her life had been...

In the middle of the night, I awoke to the sound of coughing. Standing in the doorway of the unlit room, Bubbles was gasping for breath, as she labored to take in the cool air of the night.

"I'll be alright," she insisted.

Leading her back to the couch, I sat with her until the attack passed. In between, we talked about the last days, and I reiterated my surprise at what happened between Mr. Vasquez and Jojo.

"He treated us that way," she responded. "If I ever cried, he'd thump on my chest and tell me to stop it. I had to suck in my tears."

I shook my head, disbelieving.

"I forgive him, though," she added. "I forgive my father."

74

Just then, Mr. Vasquez stormed into the room.

"Your talking is keeping your mother awake!" he shouted at Bubbles. "By leaving the door opened, you've made the house all cold! You go in the room now and sleep with your mother!...

CHAPTER FIFTY-FOUR

Getting up from the giant chair, there was a very pleasant looking restaurant across from us, and I suggested we have dinner there.

It turned out to be a Brazilian restaurant, known for serving all kinds of meat, which was interesting to her.

"I like meat," she said...

CHAPTER FIFTY-FIVE

All there was to drink was Brazilian Ginger ale. Nevertheless, she held her glass high and suggested we make a toast.

To your birthday, I said.

"And to yours," she responded...

I liked the salad bar and the cooked pineapple, mushrooms, and lobster bisque. I mostly did not like to the meat at the Brazilian restaurant. It just felt like biting into dead flesh. I suppose my attempt at the meat (which essentially amounted to trying a thimble-full before discarding it) was not unlike what I subjected her to in the pizza we'd shared in Philadelphia, when I discarded all of the cheese as a matter of maintaining my vegan obligation per my Qi Gong initiation.

"I think it's hilarious," she'd said at the time...

CHAPTER FIFTY-SIX

Bubbles described situations in which she doubted herself, like with this Hindi woman who got offended by her conversation about Jesus and the Trinity and God.

I said I was surprised, because in college, if someone didn't like something she said, she would just let it roll off her shoulders.

I remember that one creep who told me he would give me an A in First Aid, and then gave me a B. After talking with him, he left the room. Bubbles had also been present, and when I turned to her and expressed my disappointment, she responded that he was stubby, and she didn't like 'stubby guys.'

Just then, this guy pops into the room again, and points at Bubbles like he caught her in a lie.

I felt bad that he had overheard me express my disappointment; but Bubbles didn't care at all, saying that if someone puts himself in a position of deliberately overhearing something, then that's his problem.

"I guess I need to listen to my younger self," she responded to the story.

Yes, it was like she had assumed my insecurities, and now I was acting with hers...

CHAPTER FIFTY-SEVEN

Bubbles described coming to like people more. I said it had been the same for me with animals and nature.

I began by telling her about that Undergraduate Dean who suggest that I consider veterinarian school, given my high marks.

I'd responded by saying, "What? Taking care of animals? That's not important."

But now I love living among the different species that I share the planet with, as well as they're sharing their lives with us... To the point that I don't want children because I felt the world was overpopulated, and I wanted more room for animals and nature.

When I look at the companionship I received from Ini and still receive from Cat Chow, I'm filled with wonder, as well as friendship and kinship. Indeed, walking amongst different species makes me feel like Adam in the Garden of Eden, for which I'd had a vision in a past-life regression seminar.

CHAPTER FIFTY-EIGHT

"Companionship"? I thought. "Company"? I looked out at the restaurant and realized that it was not unlike the one where "the Last Supper" occurred with Nikki and recounted that story to Bubbles.

When I was five or six, my father left us.

I didn't know where. My memory from that time seemingly consisted only of sitting in the back of my mom's car, and she telling my brother and me that my father had left, and they were getting something called a 'divorce', and he wouldn't be living with us anymore.

After what felt like an eternity, my father came for my brother and me, and drove us to a downtown apartment. Inside, the apartment was poorly lit; darkly frosted mirrors lined the walls; curtains blocked the sunlight; and hanging beads in a doorway that separated the den from some interior bedroom.

Then, from behind the beads, emerged a naked woman; tall and expressionless, she towered over me like an Amazon.

I'd been sitting on the couch; as she moved past, I froze; even when my brother called out, I found myself incapable of so much as turning my head.

"Why did she do that?"

I didn't know. Perhaps, this was her way of saying, "This is my house, and – young children or not – I'm not about to change."

"Was she mean to you?"

I wouldn't say that she was 'mean' - just distant.

Sadly, the time with her that I remember best would be our last.

"What happened?"

We'd been on camping trip; the tent set near a stream; sunlight twinkled off the cool, running water; I remember its fresh taste in my mouth.

During the night we sat around a camp-fire. Other camping trips, my father had brought a short-wave radio and we'd listen to ghost stories; this time, we didn't have one, so I attempted one.

"Ugh, why do children tell such stupid stories?" Nikki said at the end of my tale.

Then, she glared at me.

"Why do you think people have children?" she said.

I shrugged.

"Maybe because they want company," I said.

She threw her head back against the log she'd been leaning, her eyes closed to the stars above.

"That's selfish!" she said. "If you want company, get a dog!..."

"But your dad liked her, right?"

I suppose, though he didn't entirely agree with the things she'd say. This was especially true the last day I'd ever see her; the four of us – my father, Nikki, my brother and I – were coming back from a hike. I remember smiling, imbued in happy thoughts of what lay ahead. Fishing! What I'd been waiting for all trip long. Now, my father had promised we'd go just as soon we got back to camp. I could hardly contain my excitement, as I ambled along.

Coming into view was a thin chain tethered between two trees on each side of the path and hanging about a foot from the ground. My brother leapt into action.

"Watch me, Dad," my brother called out. "I'm going to jump over it."

"Joe, you come back here!" my father shouted.

"Oh, let him be," Nikki responded, annoyed.

Jeff ran and leapt, but caught his toe on the chain. He tumbled in a heap, then got up, brushed himself off, and continued his merry way.

"You see," Nikki said, triumphant. "He fell. He's okay."

But my father's featured had darkened.

"Listen, when you have children of your own, you can let them run and jump and hurt themselves all you want," he said. "But these are my kids, and they'll do what I say."

"But as long as you've 'fixed' yourself," he continued, "you have nothing to say about it."

Arriving back at the campsite, I immediately set about assembling my fishing pole. Then, my father appeared and announced that we were breaking camp.

"*Why, Dad?*" *I said.*

"*Because Nikki wants to go home,*" *he responded.*

The drive felt like an eternity. Nikki's dog (named Rei, a German shepherd) sat drooling on me as the cool breeze poured in through the open window.

Finally, we stopped at what looked like a large log cabin. Inside, there was a large gathering of people; a man pleasantly conversing with another over a drink at the bar; a pleasant hostess led us between tables until seating us near a wooden stage. Nikki's features softened, as she pleasantly looked out.

"*I used to dance at a place like this,*" *she said.* "*I fell off a stage not very different from this one and hurt my leg.*"

I looked at the stage, and imagined her falling, and felt sad.

"*Is the reason you wanted to leave early because you were mad at my father for what he said to you?*" *I asked.*

"*That's part of it,*" *she said.*

I nodded and looked away, my eyes settling on a plain-looking woman at another table who sat smiling, pleasantly engaged in the conversation and friendly banter there.

I turned back to Nikki.

"*What will happen now?*" *I asked.*

"*I don't know,*" *she responded.* "*This might be our last supper...*"

Sometime after the trip, I overheard my father talking on the phone, saying that he needed to find a "home" for Rei.

"*What do you have to find a home for Rei for?*" *I asked.*

"*Because Nikki died,*" *he said, bluntly.* "*She killed herself... She took a lot of sleeping pills.*"

My mind flashed to the last time I'd seen Nikki – on that walk to the campsite – that last evening at the restaurant.

"*Was the reason that you and Nikki split up because of Joe and me?*" *I asked, timidly.*

"*That was part of it,*" *he said...*

Years later, when my mother learned about occurrences at Nikki's, she expressed disdain. I couldn't bear to hear her speak ill of Nikki, and came to her defense.

"*Well,*" *said my mother,* "*would it be okay for me to walk around naked in front of Marty's children?*"

Marty was my mother's boyfriend and male role model, with two sons the same ages as Joe and me.

No, I thought. That would be inappropriate...

I think I was perhaps 15 when it was discovered that I was harboring feelings of guilt for Nikki's death. My mother found some of my writings about nikki that I kept hidden in a space behind my dresser drawer. She told me that I shouldn't. That it wasn't my fault. I think she informed my father and we talked about it, too.

Mostly I remember how hard I wept that day. As my mother stood at the threshold of the doorway, I asked for privacy. Bowing her head, she stood there, as I closed the door. I could hear her steps as she walked away, as I sat crumpled at my desk, weeping.

Somehow, I'd become that kind of person – who doesn't take others in, in a moment of deep despair. That's when I want to be at arm's length. Arms around me are for good times. Sorrow is for alone.

In later years my father and I came to take summer trips together. In one through the Southwest I asked about Nikki and why it might have been that she took her life?

"She was a disturbed person," he said. "She'd been in counseling for years, but never could put her demons behind her."

He recalled a morning when the two of them were in the kitchen.

"Nikki said, 'Why don't we get married?'

"I considered it, but then I thought about all of her baggage and told her, 'I don't think that's such a good idea.'

"Well, as you could imagine, the relationship sort of fizzled after that.

"We stayed friends. The day before I found her, I was going to show her my new car.

"But on the way to her apartment, I got a call from work. Something came up and there were some things that I had to take care of, so I called her and told her we'd have to reschedule.

"A couple of days later, I got a call from her landlord, saying that the dog was inside barking like crazy. That's when I went over and we found her.

"Afterwards, I'd ask myself, 'What if I had gone over that day? Would it have made a difference? Could I have stopped her?...'"

It turned out that Nikki had called my father the week before her suicide.

"She was really ill," he said. "I was with Annette [my stepmother] at the time. We had just started dating then. But when I spoke to Nikki and heard how she sounded, I told Annette that I had to go over and help her.

"She said, 'Alright,' so I went to Nikki's. She looked terrible. She hadn't taken care of herself. Hadn't taken care of the dog. The place was a mess.

"So, I cleaned up the place, cooked, talked with her. I wasn't a psychiatrist. I was just trying to do what any friend would do.

"Then, after the fourth day, I get there, and the place is all cleaned up, and the table is set, and she's cooked a meal, and she's all made up, and I'm thinking to myself, 'Well, this is a change.'

"After dinner, she tells me that some guy had invited her out for the weekend, and asked what I thought she should do? I told her, 'Maybe it would be good to get out.'

"Well, you know what happened after that. The apartment manager calls me, and we found her lying on the bed. Obviously, that whole thing about being invited out for the weekend had been made up..."

He called Nikki's family.

"When I called and told them that their daughter had passed away, they just said, 'Okay, thank you,' and then hung up. Like it wasn't anything unusual. Like they expected it."

Nikki had grown up in Lido, a ranching town not far from Sacramento, California.

"She didn't talk a lot about it," he said, *"but I don't think she got along well with her parents. When she was sixteen, either she ran away or they kicked her out."*

What happened in those intervening years after that my father didn't know.

"But you can imagine that a girl with her looks probably saw a lot," he said.

I didn't ask whether he inquired if they wanted Nikki's dog? From the way it sounded, they had no interest about their daughter at all.

"The woman who answered the phone was pleasant," He said. *"Told me, 'Thank you for calling.'"*

Didn't want to know who this person was who'd called. Didn't want to know about the life she lived. Just, *"they were pleasant."* *"Told me, 'Thank you.'"* Just a being you'd supported ninie months in your womb. *"Thank you."*

What kind of parents were these?

He told me that Nikki hadn't gotten along with her parents. That she left the house young. Maybe 16.

"A girl with looks like Nikki you imagine got a lot of attention – most of it unwanted." maybe that's why she was always so angry looking? Maybe that's why she didn't typically smile? Maybe she wasn't free for that kind of thing? Maybe she had to?

"They didn't attend the funeral," he said.

My father said Nikki opened a door to a world he had not known.

"Where I grew up, it was 99% Jewish," he said. "Sure, I was poor and had to live by my wits if I was going to survive, but still my view of the world was relatively small.

"She was so different from anyone or anything I'd ever known before that."

"She made me grow up," he said. "Someone as outspoken as she was, you were either going to learn to be a man or else you weren't going to stay around."

He said that her demise did not entirely surprise him.

"She said she would never live past thirty-five," he said. "She didn't have much purpose. She was afraid of growing old. She was afraid of losing her looks.

"There were drugs involved, too. In California at that time, everyone was using marijuana, but then I went over one day and I saw this bottle of white powder, and then she's spilling it on a plate and then sniffing it into her nose. She said she only did it after breakfast before she went to work. But you know how that goes..."

CHAPTER FIFTY-NINE

Bubbles asked if I liked Nikki?

"Why not?" I responded. "She had a brain and a mind to ask difficult, thought-provoking questions: "Why do people have children?... Why do children tell such stupid stories?..."

But she didn't like kids.

I thought of the time in a park when I was trailing behind my father and his girlfriend, Nikki.

When I indicated that I was tired, Nikki turned, then hoisted me up, threw me over her shoulder and began carrying me away. To this day I can remember watching helplessly as the ground moved beneath me and feeling terrified of falling from that height.

"Let me down!" I cried. "Let me down!..."

"Like you were a burlap sack," Bubbles said, "that she just threw over her shoulder."

I talked about the difference between she and Nikki. About the experience at the Bakersfield fair with Zachary, compared to my experience with Nikki.

After donating blood at the Red Cross, Nellie, Bubbles and I drove to the County Fair. There, the Vasquez's middle daughter, Edie, was waiting with her children – an agreeable infant named Christopher and a three-year old named Zackary.

As we ventured into the fairgrounds, Zackary lagged behind. Watching him, he seemed painfully shy and sensitive, and I wondered how I or anyone could reach him to show him that the world wasn't such a fearful place and he didn't have to be so guarded and afraid?

Just then, Bubbles swooped in and hoisted the boy upon her shoulders and led him from ride-to-ride. Filled with excitement, his laughter filled the air, and watching them, I wondered that perhaps she might save him from a fear-filled childhood and infuse him with that spark of joy?

And following them through the fairgrounds, my mind wandered – confusing Liz with Bubbles, me with Zackary, as feelings and people flowed one into another...

Who was I fooling? I thought later. Of course, I didn't like Nikki. My heart broke for my mother, and Nikki was at heart of the reason that my mother was depressed. I tried to hide my feelings behind my smiley disposition, but I think on at least one occasion, they came out: It was when my father invited Joe and me to play the equivalent of 'puppy pile' with Nikki, and I wanted to hurt her.

In retrospect, I did like Nikki's body, though, even if it was traumatic to see her naked coming through those beads that first time.

Bubbles had a body like Nikki – tall and statuesque – and it occurred to me that perhaps she was my Nikki – the beautiful, risqué woman who captured my imagination, but was nice instead of distant and mean...

CHAPTER SIXTY

I told Bubbles about a young girl in the neighborhood, named Sienna, for whom every time I see her, it has the effect of brightening my day.

"I was watching her riding her bike and performing tricks on it, like standing on the seat," I said. "And watching her reminded me of the story you told me about how sad you were when your father took your bikes away... I describe that experience in my every iteration of my Bioenergy texts..."

One last experience...

I'll conclude with one final story: On a summer day my beloved college friend Bubbles and I rode out to the fields beyond the campus, and sitting under the shade of a tree sharing a picnic lunch, exchanged stories from our lives. She described the sad occurrence of a neighborhood girl struck by a drunk driver; the girl had been riding her bike at the time, and when she died, Bubbles' father reacted harshly. "He took our bikes away," Bubbles said. "We were never allowed to ride them again." She broke off and looked away. Gazing at her I knew her father had only acted to try to protect the daughters he loved! But, at the same time, I realized it made her sad.

Then, it happened: I forgot myself, and all that mattered was my cherished friend; this accompanied by a feeling like I'd left my physical body and were existing only in spirit.

"I feel for you," I said, reaching out to her. "I feel for you."

At that moment I knew who and how I was meant to be. That memory guided me to Medical Chi Healing, because every time I connected with the energetic circulation of another, I experienced that feeling. Now, I don't need to be performing Medical Chi Healing to experience that feeling, because it's become a part of me and the way I feel in general.

In sum, Medical Chi Healing is about reaching beyond oneself and connecting with another. It's about unconditional love and a way to give and receive it...

Bubbles responded that she didn't do anything they put her quite that at risk, so she described an occasion when she acquired some brand-new white sneakers, and she was so happy with those sneakers, that she found yourself looking down at them as she was riding at Top Speed, so that she wound up accidentally crashing into some railroad tracks and falling from the bike and bouncing several times along the tracks.

"And all I remember of it was just calling out, 'Ouch... Ouch... Ouch...'"

It made me think of the time that the train was parked in front of the street for several minutes, so that several athletic fellas were just tossing their bikes onto the train and then crossing to the other side of the train; However, when I finally decided to do that, too, naturally, the train started moving, so I was left to jump off of this moving train and hurt my back...

CHAPTER SIXTY-ONE

She said that she thought she could be more unconditionally loving.

I nodded, though I couldn't imagine her having been more unconditionally loving towards me. She was my "gold standard" where that was concerned...

CHAPTER SIXTY-TWO

She went to the salad bar.

Arriving back at the table, she said, "As I was walking back, I thought, 'I like seeing you at the table and the thought of spending more time talking with you.'"

She sat.

"I liked looking at you," she added, "and seeing you there…"

CHAPTER SIXTY-THREE

Bubbles asked if I still ski? I said it depended on my friend Sam, for whom I develop such a fondness for his skiing that I preferred to watch him ski than ski myself.

"Just to watch him cut through that snow at blinding speed," I said. "It's amazing - Sam's grace on skis is a thing of beauty."

At 70 years old, he was encountering quite a bit of pain, though, and problems in his body were keeping him from skiing, so that I wasn't skiing as much because he wasn't going up with me.

Then, it struck me that I had never personally told her about my skiing before, and it must have been she'd learned about it by reading my letters.

And then it occurred to me that the last time we had been together was when I visited her in Las Vegas 16 years ago - The visit that she couldn't remember.

Just the other day, April and I had been talking about how it was that she and ROBERT would have these cycles in which they'd go in and out of interacting with each other, and where she was feeling so terrible about not having been there for him at the time of his death, because she'd been in one of those cycles after this obnoxious thing he done by sending her a text with a antisemitic comment.

At the time, I'd reminded April that she'd told me she'd expected Bubbles not to interact with me for perhaps as long as 20 years given the way I'd responded to her sending me an obituary about her father a year after he died, without any comment.

"Yeah, it only took 16 years," April had said...

CHAPTER SIXTY-FOUR

Bubbles asked about other physical activities I was engaging in?
"I remember you used to throw a mean bowling ball," she said.

I hesitated. I couldn't remember even once going bowling with her. Yet, she could remember bowling after 40 years ago and not remember my most recent visit.

It must have happened when we were still living in the dorms, because we didn't go bowling during our summers together – That I would have remembered.

I wondered why she would remember a time when we were in the dorms and before we were intimate?

Or was the reason why she remembered that because she was in love with me even before our summer together?

"I've always loved you, David…"

In the dorms, I was in love with Terry Mehta - The other angel on the dorms. The only woman whose beauty could rival Bubbles.

Indeed, after the summer with Bubbles, I asked Terry out… But compared to what I had with Bubbles, there was nothing there. It was like an intellectual exercise. There was none of the connection and fun and intimacy like I had with Bubbles.

Of note, Terry knew that Bubbles loved me when the three of us were living in the dorms, because I'd told Terry about how Bubbles helped me overcome my despair over a mistake I'd made in the lab.

It happened this way: I created a computer problem for scientific mentor, Prof. Hope. He cursed at me – "Dave! Fuck you, Dave. Get out of here! Go home!" I left there feeling crushed; I thought my dreams of a career in science had gone up in smoke, and felt so ashamed that I remained hunkered in my dorm room, feeling I'd never recover from what I'd done.

For days, the only time I'd leave the room was for meals at the Dining Commons. That's where Bubbles saw me from clear across the Commons, in spite of hundreds of other students in between us.

"I think there's something's wrong with Dave," she told Jim.

"Oh, he's probably just mad at me again," Jim responded.

"No, I think it's something different," she insisted.

She was sitting at the end of our usual dormitory communal table (whereas I'd been consuming my meal alone at a smaller table). As I was making my way out of the Commons, she looked up at me, smiling.

"How you doing, Davy?" she asked.

"Not good, Bubbles," I said, my head bowed and shaking.

"What's the matter?" she asked.

I hesitated, then responded, "I can't tell you", completely uncharacteristic and contrary to any way I'd ever been.

I left then and went back to my room. Not long after, though, to my surprise, there was a knock at my door. When I opened it, Bubbles walked past me into the interior of my room (Something she'd never done) and then, paced back and forth.

"Dave, you've got to tell me what's the matter," she insisted. "You've got to tell me what you're feeling."

I nodded and said I'd tell her if she'd accompany across the street to the market. She came and we talked, and then she came back to my room and sat on the bed and comforted me, until she'd chased all my dark clouds away and replaced them with skies of blue.

And then, she held me and told me that she loved me, and kissed me on the neck, so to send chills all through me.

I written a poem about it, and shared it with Terry.

"Would you consider more with Bubbles?" Terry asked after I'd read the poem.

"No!" I responded, unhesitatingly. "She's with Jim!"

But Terry knew. She knew Bubbles loved me. It was just me who didn't.

Saturday, May 12, 1984
After a day with Bubbles.

Bubbles, you have so much love, so much love for me,
Sometimes, when I look deeply into your eyes, I feel myself just melt,
Melt in your love and the warm feeling you kindle inside of me.

Bubbles, you kiss me gently on my neck, on my cheek, and then embrace me with your entire body against mine.
You tell me you love me,
You tell me you're glad for me,
You tell me you enjoyed temple and that we'll have to go again soon.
I say I love you, too.
I tell you you're wonderful and how much I enjoy spending time with you.

Bubbles, you give me such a wonderful feeling down deep inside.
You make me feel like I am beautiful.
You supersede my intensity and bring out a feeling of tranquility and love for life.

Bubbles, I feel for you so much.
Life is hard for you, yet you still smile.
Sometimes, I feel helpless, knowing how much I want to help and how hard life can be on a person.

Bubbles, you're an angel.
But for some reason,
I don't know why,
You seem to be an angel born for toil and endurance of life's hardships.
Oh, why, oh, why, so much the victim of love's cruelty?

Bubbles, I do love you.
When you take me in your arms,
I feel myself sinking gently, tenderly into love's grip.
You make me feel alive.
You make me feel loved.

Bubbles, stay with me.
Don't become another casualty in life's game of moving on.
You, your love, means so much to me.
The time I spend with you is time made to stand still,
To bring out in me life's joy,
To make me to see how good life really is,
To make me see how much I love,
How much I love you, Bubbles,
And how much you love me.

In retrospect, I think that might have been an energy experience Bubbles had back then: When she knew something was wrong with me from across that crowded cafeteria, I think it was because she picked up on a disturbance in my energetic circulation.

And then came to my room and insisted I talk to her.

Because, for whatever reason, she loved me...

CHAPTER SIXTY-FIVE

Bubbles told me that of the choices I'd given her for lunch for our prior plans on Friday, she'd chosen the Ethiopian restaurant because she used to eat Ethiopian food while she was attending Veterinarian School in Fort Collins, Colorado.

When I couldn't make it because I was still attending my mother's affairs, I said I'd pay for lunch at the restaurant; however, she said she didn't wind up going, because her son had a "tummyache" and didn't want to chance eating something different before the band event, which she regarded as a smart decision on his part...

CHAPTER SIXTY-SIX

By the 2nd to 3rd hour at the Brazilian restaurant, we'd mostly run out of things to say.

She inquired why I was looking into the distance?

"Is it because you think it's safe for you to breathe the air with your head turned further to the outside?" she asked.

No, I said. It's because I was enjoying the image of her in my peripheral vision.

She looked at me quizzically, so I continued by telling her that it was until relatively late in my childhood that it was determined that I had significant nearsightedness.

"Basically," I said. "I found out in junior high school because I was fooling around with a friend's glasses one day and tell him that all of his sudden, I could see everything crystal clear on the chalkboard?

"I couldn't have imagined that in my wildest dreams. I just thought when things were further away, you couldn't see them... That it was just natural that they become blurry. And now, here I was with my friend's glasses on, and I could see everything crystal clear?

"To this day, I still remember the first thing I saw with my new glasses: It was the night sky, and being able to see all of those stars so clearly for the first time in my life was utterly amazing to me.

"But wearing them at school, I was overwhelmed: It was so different to be in that kind of world where you could see the expression on everybody's face all the way across the hall 100 feet away. It all felt like too much for a sensitive kid like me."

"I can imagine how that was traumatic," she interjected.

"So, I find a sense of ease and comfort in my blurry world," I concluded.

Then, I asked if she minded me just looking at her, even if I didn't have things to say?

"No, I don't mind," she said.

I looked at her, taking in her great beauty; but, then, found myself looking into the distance and keeping her in my peripheral vision.

I figured it was just a habit.

But perhaps there was more to it? Perhaps it was because her beauty was still too blinding for me?

Really, given what we'd been to each other, how could I look at her, with her smiling eyes, without being moved and moving to kiss her?

My mind drifted to discussions I'd had with Native American Medicine Men when it came to energy healing practices. It turned out that their approach was similar to mine, with one significant exception: According to them, it was always practiced with eyes closed. For them, practicing it with eyes open was taboo.

I remembered how it was that she would ask why I always kept my eyes closed when I kissed her? I said it was because I just wanted to appreciate the sensation of her lips on mine, and not any other senses.

And with that, I smiled, feeling I could understand my Medicine Men colleagues in their insistence in performing energy healing the way they did.

With that, I felt inspired to sing a Lakota prayer song and asked her if I could share it?

Du way waka-ta waka, Cha che waki ey lo hi.
Ti wa hey ki, Dy ya namach hu we lo hey yo.

I explained its meaning:

For all that is sacred, I drum and sing.
For all of creation, I am grateful.

"I think of you," I told her...

CHAPTER SIXTY-SEVEN

We talked about dreams, and I reminded her that when we were together, she said she was always being killed in them.

"I'm always killed in my dreams," she said upon awakening from one of them. "Most of the time I get an ax thrown into my back - That's why my back gets sore."

"Oh, I remember how the dream started now," she continued. "You and I were making love."

"I was in the dream?" I asked.

"Yeah," she replied. "We were making love. Then you said, 'Come on, Bubbles' and I followed you into a tunnel, and you disappeared, and I was in this train..."

I'd felt guilty about that dream, like my transient presence in her life was the source of the nightmare, and that's where my love had taken her, and perhaps I could have made a difference by staying with her?

Oddly, though, it struck me that while I was caring for her mother before her mother's open-heart surgery, I'd had a dream that amounted to my letting myself die by seemingly willingly falling to my death.

Climbing a jagged mountain, I labored to propel myself upwards. At the top I saw Bubbles standing and following the progress of my ascent.

Then, rounding the final turn between two spires at the peak, I closed my eyes, leaned back and let myself go falling back to the earth without fear...

Why in the world would I have voluntarily decided to lean back and fall to my death? I thought now.

I shook my head.

It made no sense, I decided.

Anyway, I guess she wasn't the only one with dreams of dying?...

Earlier in the day, I'd told her about the very pleasant dream I'd last had about her.

"I went to hold you," I recounted. "But I was holding so tightly that you squealed and called out, 'David, my chest.'"

She'd smiled.

"That was a good dream," I concluded...

CHAPTER SIXTY-EIGHT

It was close to 10, and Bubbles had to pick up her son.

I paid the bill for dinner, and we walked to our cars.

I had my mask back on and told her that I'd like to take it off to kiss her before she left.

But when I did, rather than kiss me, she pecked me? Or maybe the reason it felt like it was because her lips had grown so thin?

In any event, unlike any other time that she'd ever kissed me, there wasn't the 'fireworks' like there'd always been before. Even that first time when we were just friends and she saw me all down and depressed after Professor Hope cursed at me and she insisted I had to tell her what was the matter and what I was feeling, and before she left my room, after pulling me out of my despair, she kissed me on the neck, and that kiss flooded my system with such a rush of endorphins as to send chills up and down my spine and through my whole body. And then, with every kiss since – until this one.

I thought about the day after we first attempted intimacy, when she came to the lab, and it was just the most natural thing in the world to approach her, kiss her, as though our bodies should merge with each other, were meant to merge with each other, every atom intertwine.

I wondered if it was because she had to hold herself back?

I thought about 40 years ago, when she came back from Bakersfield, and I showed her my new apartment, and while I went to get something for us to drink, she sat on the floor, and I was overcome with admiration for her – her grace and humility - I fell to my knees and hold her; and she reciprocated, because she said she wanted to share her feelings with me.

And now she wasn't doing that.

It just seemed like she/we have been taken away from your 'true nature.'

Even in Philadelphia, she told me that she loved me before parting...

But it seems she was also closed emotionally, so that that connection was blocked when I kissed her.

"I think she was being defensive," a psychology colleague said. "What I'm hearing is defensiveness, saying to you, 'You haven't moved on.' She's not talking about the two of you. She's just looking at you. It's like she has a lot of barriers to you..."

Thirty years ago, she was blocked when it came to bioenergy; today, she was blocking her feelings.

"She's conflicted because part of her knows not to get involved," my friend, Reuben, asserted. "Because the truth is, if you guys did get involved, it's a big mess! And it's going to affect people other than yourselves. You both have commitments to others now..."

CHAPTER SIXTY-NINE

"So, she's changed," my therapist would comment later.

I thought she was just doing the best she could: She smiled and invited me to sit with her and look upon her, but putting an arm around her or kissing her was off-limits.

"Yeah, it sounds like a lot of mixed messages," she continued. "It's hard to be with someone like that."

Again, what could she do – especially where it was so easily for me to, as Nietzsche would say, become overcome with 'madness in love' for her.

In what she was willing to give, I'd enjoyed my time being lost with her. There was just the joy of being with her. I wasn't thinking of anything I had to do. There wasn't any place I particularly wanted to go. All I wanted to do was be with her. She is the one person for whom just being in her presence is enough – And it doesn't matter where we are or what we're doing. I am doing what I want by just being with her. Because of the way it triggers my endorphins system or energetic circulation or whatever.

And I learned something: That her kisses – They hadn't come from her lips - at least, not the ones I was looking for – They'd come from her heart. Those were the only kind of kisses from her I wanted. The ones that elicit the fireworks. I didn't want the other ones, because they just diminish the memory of the first. Even if I never kissed her again…

CHAPTER SEVENTY

Before departing, I asked if I could give her an insulated bag in the shape of a picnic basket in acknowledgement of all the times she'd come around to the lab with her picnic basket full of bagels to see that I had something to eat during our summer together.

As she was about to leave, she indicated that her son would probably participate in the Claireville band event again and need to be chaperoned, so we could probably meet this way next year...

CHAPTER SEVENTY-ONE

Watching her pull away, it felt to an extent like the visit started the way it began: She looked frozen in the beginning when she pulled up in her car, and now she looked frozen as she left. Like she was perhaps preparing herself to not be herself and cut herself off from her feelings and sharing those feelings.

In that way, it was worse than in Philadelphia, because at least there she came out of herself for a brief moment to tell me that she loved me too before I got on the train...

CHAPTER SEVENTY-TWO

"Did it leave you with feelings of regret?" April asked. "Or did you feel more reconciled?"

It was just a joy to be with her.

And feeling like we are still friends who love each other, perhaps even deeper than we had at any other time.

And I appreciated her permitting me to expressed my issues of non-closure and not being harsh or judgmental towards me...

CHAPTER SEVENTY-THREE

Returning from Claireville, I stepped out of the truck at my usual parking spot and found myself surrounded by thick, green vegetation that displaced and seemingly swallowed up all the building that had been previously standing nearby, as though a thousand years had passed between when I'd left and when I got back there?...

Awakening from the dream, I interpreted it to mean that, in the span of those few hours with Bubbles, a world had happened.

That and I was caught in an energetic feeling of being intimate with Bubbles, so that I felt her at my loins and imagined this was a manifestation of her feelings reaching out to me, not unlike the energy experience I'd had all those years ago after caring for her mother:

The bus drove off; but instead of the familiar emptiness and hollowness in my chest, another sensation filled me: It was a feeling of energy, starting at my head, then beaming and overflowing to every part of me – Till I was immersed and enveloped in what felt like a cocoon of energy, fuller and more expansive than anything I'd ever experienced before.

I've honored something, I thought. I've shown some great respect. It relates to something simple, yet wonderful, and reaches to the core of my being.

The bus drove on into the night and the feeling continued to radiate. Resting, my body conformed to the contours of the seat, as I breathed easy and felt the onset of sleep.

I want to hang on to this feeling, but I have to trust that tomorrow is another day. This connection I feel – a connection to a higher source. It radiates from my head upwards – God is love...

CHAPTER SEVENTY-FOUR

I texted Bubbles:

Me: I so enjoyed spending the day with you. Thank you.

She: I enjoyed your company as well. Thank you for speaking freely with me.

Me: I know you told me you wanted to spend the day studying about performing ultrasounds, but could I interest you in some more of my bioenergy/Qi Gong services for at least a little while? Perhaps I can also bring you bagels and lox for breakfast or something from the Ethiopian restaurant for lunch?

She: That's a long drive for a short time. Last year Taylor was done before 5pm. Our flight boards at 7pm. Maybe then?

Me: The drive matters to me not at all. If you think bioenergy/Qi Gong would be helpful and if you'd like me to bring some food, I would be more than happy – overjoyed! – to do so...

CHAPTER SEVENTY-FIVE

I bought bagels, cream cheese and lox, and waited. But Bubbles didn't reach back, except to text a selfie she'd taken of the two of us from yesterday on the giant chair…

CHAPTER SEVENTY-SIX

April indicated that she'd been nervous about my having stayed out so late with Bubbles.

"Because if she were available, you'd be with her," she said.

But would I? Would I give up pursuing my ability to be free to follow my callings in life? It was hard for me to imagine. The lack of closure in our relationship was eating me alive, such that no one else could be good enough for me or compare; but having made that choice forty years ago, my life was my own, and I could live it as I pleased.

Nevertheless, when I considered the crippling changes suggested by the outlines of her feet, it did trouble me. Then, I wanted to turn my head away, as it was too much for me to take in.

"You want to be there for her," Reuben responded, spiritedly. "You want to be there this way for her, I know. You were probably just blown away, thinking, 'I should be sending her to doctors. And if not that, I want to be doing it myself. I want to be her doctor. I want to be her friend. I want to help her remember. I want this life with her.'"

"But can you go there?" he asked. "Can she go there? You would have to sacrifice a great deal to go there. Can you do that?"

'Sacrifice', I thought. Yes, she was the sacrifice. A life with her was what I'd sacrificed for a career in medicine and science.

In the tradition of native peoples, every gift bestowed by the Creator required a sacrifice.

Hence, I'd been gifted the realizations of my dreams for science and humanity: The development of a cancer vaccine; the pursuit of research in Energy Medicine (Indeed, the Qi Gong project that I'd been leading before spending the day with her would wind up being successful beyond my wildest dreams!) – in exchange for a life with her.

And she'd sacrificed her health by going down the path she'd chosen – Because I didn't think she'd have feet like that if she'd put herself first.

Thinking about the Lakota and their tradition of honoring those spirits who'd chosen a difficult path, I thought they'd consider hers a spirit to be honored?...

CHAPTER SEVENTY-SEVEN

I told Reuben about our so-called kiss and how I faulted myself for having not recognized that on all those other occasions it was she who initiated them, and now having to live with a last kiss that was without the 'fireworks' of all the others.

"Nothing is ever a mistake when it comes to something like that," he responded, compassionately.

"Look at the truth," he continued. "Bubbles has always been someone who your heart has gone back to. Your heart wants to experience what you've never been able to experience with anyone else except her.

"And I totally understand that - You can't help feeling that way. When Sheli and I got together, we pretty much dropped everything. We felt like, 'This is my life path now. This is it.' It felt right. It felt real. It was what my life path was this time around.

"And it's tough to say, 'This time around', because I felt like we've known each other in many multiple lives. And in this one, we've tried to make it right.

"But that said, I don't think I've ever heard you say that you love anyone else but Bubbles – At least, not with the same kind of depth.

"But I've also known that in this life, even right now, you have choices. And if you were to get back together, there are consequences to it. Big consequences. And you both have to be willing to deal with those consequences. You can't go halfway. It's one of those things that you have to be all in on, or not at all. It's a full life commitment. Because there are other people involved.

"If she was totally in love with her husband, you wouldn't feel like there was any kind of chance or hope or anything with Bubbles."

Later, I would be struck by a passage from an article in the New York Times titled, "She Met Hunter Biden One Night at a Club. Then She Fell in Love", about Zoë Kestan's affair with Hunter.

In the spring of 2019, Ms. Kestan reached out to Mr. Biden to congratulate him on his daughter's high school graduation, which she had seen on Instagram. When she didn't hear back, she sent him another message to make sure he was OK. Shortly after, Mr. Biden wrote to her for the last time.

"Hi Zoe," Mr. Biden wrote in an email. "I got married to the love of my life, and I'm happier than I have ever been. I have begun a new life with my beautiful wife and ask you to please honor my privacy. Wish you well."

At first, I thought that Hunter's response was cold; but, later, to Reuben's point, I realized that if Bubbles had sent me such a text, I probably would have let her alone.

Instead, she sends me a text inviting me to spend time with her with her son?

Wherever talk goes is fine with me...

CHAPTER SEVENTY-EIGHT

"If you were totally in love with anyone else, you wouldn't be feeling the pangs of it every time you meet her and talk to her," Reuben continued. "I know this is the deepest matter of your heart. I've known this for a long time. You're someone who wants to love with all your heart someone else. You want the soulmate. You want to have the twin flame.

"And yet, you have something else that you're committed to. And her, too."

Yes, it was in her kiss. That's why it wasn't a mistake, like Reuben said. She was telling me that she can't be there physically for me anymore. No matter how much I might love her, no matter how much my heart might reach out to her, no matter how much my heart might belong to her, and no matter how much it might be she feels all those ways for me, she simply can't be there for me that way.

"I believe you guys will get another shot at it," Reuben continued, "but, more than likely, not in this lifetime, but the next.

"My only advice to you is, if you love her, love her.

"And it's the truth. You do. You love her.

"So, love her. That's fine.

"Will you live a life together right now, probably not. Might you in the future? Who knows?

"It's much more complicated now than it was forty years ago – for both of you - were it to happen now..."

CHAPTER SEVENTY-NINE

But where does my love for her go? I wondered. Was it really just a matter of you love and you die carrying such feelings in your heart?

April commented about my day with Bubbles by describing what an experience with Ini had taught her, referencing Ini's last joyful day at the park.

"We had spent hours in the park," she began. "And then you came around and we were all surrounding her, and Ima has a picture of it, and Ini was very joyful. She was so happy. We were all happy.

"So, I know she suffered up to that point – and that she continued to suffer afterwards – But if we think she was willing to suffer to be with us… Well, she had that moment - She was really, really happy then…"

April became tearful.

"You can't always expect tomorrow," she continued. "And the really, really important thing, especially if you're having a joyful moment with someone that you love and want to be with me, is to just be with that moment of joy. You stay with it. You treasure it. You remember it. You honor it.

"And if you have something you have to do later, then you change it. You just go, 'Now is the moment. Now, everything is aligned. I am having an amazing moment with a person I love, and I'm not going to take it for granted, and I am just going to be thoroughly in it. This is what makes all the suffering worth it. This moment… So, I'm just going to take it, and be with it, and memorialize it. This is what life's about.'

"And this comes from my regret about not grabbing that moment of joy with Ini and just staying with you in the park. And then when it started raining, just go running out of the park. But first, be in that moment with her - And not expect another moment later, or even think about making her something to eat or something like that. Just be like, 'This is why she is still here, and I'm not going to take it for granted it. I'm just going to be with it.'

"That's a regret I have, and I'm going to try not to have that regret again with somebody else I love - Though I am forever going to treasure that moment with Ini that Wednesday afternoon.

"So, in terms of Bubbles, I think, treasure yesterday and savor it. If it happens again, then it happens again. But that's a gift. And just treasure it.

"Her life is complicated. Your life is complicated. People are connected to you and to her.

"So just treasure those hours you had together..."

EPILOGUE

Taylor was here last week. He told me that he does not need me to travel with him to CA next month. HE DOESN'T NEED ME ANYMORE 😦 😦 *Not that he said that harshly, just that he is growing up....*
I am very proud of him, making his way in the world. I know I spoke to you about this before; my heart and mind is saddened by the circle of life. As if I thought the world could stand still for me...give me more time...let me be refreshed and live in the moment instead of toiling to provide...

As the text from Bubbles indicated, there was no returning to Claireville the following year.

"And because of her possessive husband, she can never just go on a reunion trip and see you?" my friend, Steve, asked.

No. I'd indicated to her that I wanted that, but she hadn't responded.

"I'm just sorry that you're not going to see each other," he replied, sadly, "for probably ever."

Yes, whereas her son had moved towards autonomy and independence, she was still in my endorphin system and likely always would be.

Confiding my sadness to my friend, Sam, he responded this way:

"Getting lost and stuck in the past is easy to do," he began. "It requires energy to move out of that."

118

"I mean it's good to enjoy that and have that, but not to be chained to it," he continued. "And, so, you have to put in some energy to break the chain and move forward.

"Because being in the present is important – and also the future. More important than being in the past.

"Probably most important is how do you divide your time? Put 15% of your energy in the past. And 70% in the present. And another 15% into the future – because you can't ignore the future, because the future will eventually become the present – and then the past. So, the more you can mold the future, you can have a more predictable present and past.

"I keep on thinking - when I think of you - you have a vision for the future for yourself. And I think you just need to focus and get some more clarity to it, so that when it becomes the present, you can make greater opportunities from it.

"One of the things to get that energy to get out of the past is to find something in the past that you can stand on. It's like Newton Third Law: Tor every action, there's an equal and opposite reaction. So, therefore, to be able to jump forward or higher, you have to be standing on something."

Yes, I was standing on her belief in me. I was standing on her desire to see me succeed in all of my dreams. I could see her showing me the way when it came to the energy of love. Like she did on that day when we were having that picnic lunch, and I experienced that feeling of being outside of myself and feeling for another for the first time - So that I recognized that feeling when I encountered it again in Bioenergy.

I believe she gifted that to me: The motivation and inspiration to embrace Bioenergy; the BioEnerQi self-practice that I'd developed based on the experience after caring for her mother, which had been so helpful to those who participated in the University of California-Davis Long COVID-Qi Gong study, which was found to impart statistically significant improvements to long COVID sufferers for problems of fatigue, pain, activity tolerance, shortness of breath, anxiety and depression. I could stand on that and take that into the future - By honoring her gift to me when it came to these things.

"So, I would say, go into the past to get something that you can stand on," Sam continued. "So that once you could stand on something, you could deal with the present in a more stable manner, and that will also allow you to leap off a bit into the future. So that the purpose of your past is to go back and get something that you had stored away that you can use. Because you kept it there for future use. And so your past has a value for your present and for your future, and that's how the relationship with the past is.

"Or else the past has all kinds of stuff, and you can be a hoarder who never finds anything that you specifically want in an efficient and timely manner – So that you can go back and get something of value, and keep your past organized, so that you can find things quicker and better that you need.

"Because that's what memories are for. And that's what dreams are for. To help you organize the value of your past, so that you can deal with the present and future in a more constructive, productive and efficient manner.

"And it brings joy! Because you didn't lose the past. In fact, you are incorporating it, so that it has a greater part and value to you for the present and future. And so it helps shape who you are. And, therefore the past creates who you are today."

"Again, when I think of you, I think you have such a bright future," he asserted. "Very few people have futures they can actually use. It's like a rope: Somebody dropped a rope for you, and that's the future. And that rope allows you to climb higher. You just need to know how to climb up the rope. That's all.

"Again, very few people have a rope to the future that is dropped down for them to use to go higher. Most people find that they have no future."

I thought of my father and his loss of executive function and persistent cognitive decline. The night before, he kept on talking about wanting to fly a plane again, and all the joy that gave him in the past, but he doesn't have the faculties to be able to engage that activity anymore.

"They have no rope," Sam declared.

"And then there are some people who use that rope to hang themselves," he continued. "Because they don't take opportunities with the rope, or because they don't use it properly. So, you have to decide how you're going to use that rope."

I think I'll climb it to a brighter place, I thought.

"Nothing is 100%," he concluded. "And a lot of it is dependent on what you do with it..."

I'd been visiting with my father at the time. There'd been a snowstorm over the past days, and, upset about my father's deteriorating condition (dementia) and the state of affairs of my life, I went aimlessly walking into the storm and climbing up a mountain. Then, struggling to ascend the snow-covered peak, I recalled the dream I'd had while caring for Bubbles' mother before she underwent open-heart surgery: I'd dreamt I was climbing a jagged mountain and laboring to propel myself upwards; at the top I saw Bubbles, standing and following the progress of my ascent; then, rounding the final turn between two spires at the peak, I closed my eyes, leaned back and let myself go falling back to the earth, without fear.

I hadn't comprehended what the dream meant thirty years ago, but now I understood perfectly: Bubbles showed me heaven; but I had to return to earth to achieve what I was put here for.

These thoughts were reinforced when, about a month later, my beloved friend and teacher, Sam, had to be hospitalized for shortness of breath. I was in the room with him when a couple of doctors entered and, like some angels of death, delivered what amounted to a death sentence to him, declaring that his condition was terminal and there was essentially nothing they could do.

And how did Sam respond to that? By caring about others. By caring about me and my future Qi Gong endeavors. Despite facing his mortality and a terrible agonizing death of worsening, worsening shortness of breath and represented my worst nightmare.

Talking that night together, Sam's energy reminded me of Bubbles. Like her, he was always a person who I considered too good for this world. Always treating people with so much kindness, and, somehow, he could ignore that that kindness wasn't reciprocated. Who always gave a kind, warm, supportive, healing energy to everyone. Like Bubbles would shower on me.

Falling asleep, I dreamt of Bubbles: We were back at the University and made our way to the back patio of a house somewhere, and behind some curtains, we pulled each other clothes and kiss the way we used to.

Awakening from that dream, I experienced a feeling of emptiness in my chest, and went back to wondering about having known heaven with Bubbles, and whether that's where I'll go when I enter that morphine-assisted dream space when my life ends?...

"... angel born for toil..."

On the evening of Easter Sunday, I dreamt that I was getting around on a hover board that that belonged to Bubbles. Returning the board, I wasn't expecting her to be around at the co-ed communal home where she was living; however, she was there, and greeting me at the door in a bathrobe and towel, she invited me inside. There, we sat opposite each other in the open structure (people walking freely in the background) and she told me to please text her.

"It happens that you have been on my mind," I continued in my text about the dream, "especially as pertains to your comment about 'toiling to provide.' I've been wanting to offer to help (as I still help Kate's youngest daughter, Alyssa, to help pay for her education), but had been holding back due to the thought that the offer wouldn't be greeted well, and it wasn't my place. Now, here I am acting on the dream..."

She didn't respond. When I consider the reason, my thoughts harkened back to our summer together, and the day she'd been away on a field trip to Marineland, and I returned to the room late that night to find she still wasn't there. In the bed my mind was filled with insecurities and apprehensions, as I lay for hours, unable to sleep.

Finally, I heard some rustling in the bathroom, then the turning of the doorknob.

"Hi David," she whispered.

She sat beside me and told me about her day. The trip to Marineland had not gone as she'd anticipated, and she hadn't got what she wanted from the visit. She indicated that she was ambitious that way and added that she wanted something from everyone.

What do you want from me? I asked, timidly.
"Your love!" she'd responded, spiritedly...
Maybe it's still that way, and she's as stuck as I am?...

Where Bubbles had declared I'd lived an 'interesting life', I
hold that the reason all came back to her and the summer we
spent together: After letting her go so to pursue my dreams,
there was no ordinary life for me; at every turn in my career,
when I'd have the opportunity to settle on an ordinary life, my
thoughts returned to her, and I'd take the harder road – towards
developing a cancer vaccine or pioneering studies in Energy
Medicine; because if what I'd wanted was an ordinary life, I
would have fought like hell to make it with her.

April had urged me to write a book called *Driven.*

"About what drives you?" she said. "Why it isn't enough
for you to be just a good, caring doctor?"

I think the answer to her question is clear: Like Achilles left
Deidamia to achieve eternal glory on the fields of Troy, letting
go of Bubbles was always going to propel me towards striving
for the extraordinary.

Now, Bubbles had to do what she needed in this world,
and so did I.

She has to keep going, as a mother and as a wife.

And I have to do what I was put in this world for, as a
scientist and a healer...

At a certain point during Sam's hospitalization, I couldn't
get my mind off of him, to the point that he became my entire
focus, so that it was getting in the way of completing the
scientific manuscript about the Long Covid-Qi Gong study.

When I shared this with Carl and April, April (who is a
descendant of psychoanalysts who personally worked with
Sigmund and Anna Freud) offered the following theory:

"It makes me think about one of Dave's biggest gripes
when it comes to his dad," she said. "That when he was in
college, and he met Bubbles, and his dad was like, 'You need to
concentrate on your studies. That's more important than a girl.
You'll find girls some other time, but, right now, you should be

focueing on your etudies.' And later on, Dave wanted to build a life with her, but it was too late, so that's part of the regret."

"But I would trust Dave to know what he needs," she continued. "I know that some people can get into an eddy and focus on others, and not take care of their needs. But I also think that it's way early for that. I mean, it's only been a week. And I try to trust his judgment. and if there's something important to Dave…"

The following day, I shared my concerns with Sam, and he told me not to worry about him so much, and that he had supportive family, and I shouldn't let my concerns for him keep me from going to Yale.

Forty years ago, at a similar junction, Bubbles treated me with similar grace.

"Bubbles, you tell me: Is there any way it could work between you and me? Is there any way I could still have you and my studies and my research? Tell me, Bubbles, and I'll try. Just tell me, and I'll do everything I can."

She thought for a long time, our eyes never leaving each other.

"David, I don't think there's any way we could make it."

I lowered my head to her chest.

"I know," I said. "I just could see myself - Trying to study; trying to take time to be with you; trying to continue my research - and doing a half-ass job of all of it. I'm sorry, Bubbles. I love you. I swear I do. I love you more than anyone else in the world. But my studies come first. I just can't make the commitment."

She reached out and held my head in her hands and pulled it close to her chest.

"I know," she said. "I love you, too. But I know that in the end, you would probably be angry and despise me for being in your life…"

As with most all things, she was unquestionably right; but I have missed her. Just like I told her in a dream from long ago, "You are to me, God's greatest gift…"

ABOUT THE AUTHOR

David Fischer, M.D., Ph.D. is a physician-scientist whose groundbreaking research at the National Institutes of Health (NIH) was the basis for an FDA-approved vaccine for cancer. Following a traumatic leg injury, he was treated and trained in Bioenergy and Qi Gong. He introduced Energy Medicine approaches at the National Institute of Complementary and Integrative Health and worked with Qi Gong Masters on the President's Executive Committee on Alternative Medicine. In 2023 Dr. Fischer was the recipient of the coveted Science of Tai Chi & Qigong Award from Harvard University for his work using external Qi Gong to assist Veterans with problems of severe traumatic brain injury & neurologic deficits, chronic pain & opioid dependence, as well as long COVID & RSV. At the University of California-Davis, he led a clinical study that demonstrated the successful use of Qi Gong in the treatment of long COVID. Within the VA, he serves homeless Veterans, as well as leads efforts to combat the opioid crisis and advance integrative therapies for the treatment of pain and addiction.

www.ingramcontent.com/pod-product-compliance
Lightning Source LLC
Chambersburg PA
CBHW060504280326
41933CB00014B/2854